Asthma - Diagnosis, Management and Comorbidities

Edited by Öner Özdemir

Published in London, United Kingdom

Asthma - Diagnosis, Management and Comorbidities
http://dx.doi.org/10.5772/intechopen.1008593
Edited by Öner Özdemir

Contributors
Gabriel Román-Ríos, Guzin Ozden, Katarzyna Napiórkowska-Baran, Leyla Cevirme, Mehmet Kılıç, Nasrin Fazel, Patricia Silveyra, Ricardo A. Mosquera, Shima Rasouli, Stefan-Marian Frent, Wilfredo De Jesús-Rojas, Yosima Gonzalez, Öner Özdemir

First published in London, United Kingdom, 2025 by IntechOpen
IntechOpen is the global imprint of INTECHOPEN LIMITED, registered in England and Wales, registration number: 11086078, 167-169 Great Portland Street, London, W1W 5PF, United Kingdom

For EU product safety concerns: IN TECH d.o.o., Prolaz Marije Krucifikse Kozulić 3, 51000 Rijeka, Croatia, info@intechopen.com or visit our website at intechopen.com.

British Library Cataloguing-in-Publication Data
A catalogue record for this book is available from the British Library

Asthma - Diagnosis, Management and Comorbidities
Edited by Öner Özdemir
p. cm.
Print ISBN 978-1-83635-325-6
Online ISBN 978-1-83635-324-9
eBook (PDF) ISBN 978-1-83635-326-3

Meet the editor

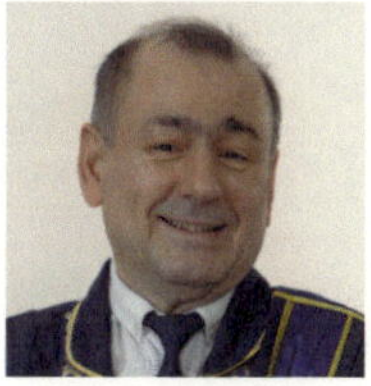

Prof. Dr. Öner Özdemir graduated from İstanbul Medical School, İstanbul University, Türkiye, and became a medical doctor in 1989. He completed his pediatric residency in the Department of Pediatrics, Children's Hospital, İstanbul Medical School, Türkiye. He completed his clinical fellowship training in the Pediatric Allergy/Immunology Division at Louisiana State University Health Sciences Center, USA. A portion of his clinical fellowship training was completed at the Pediatric Allergy/Immunology program at Cincinnati Children's Hospital Medical Center in the United States. Dr. Özdemir was the first-place winner of the 2005 Clemens Von Pirquet Award from the American College of Allergy, Asthma and Immunology (ACAAI) for the best research on allergy/asthma/immunology by a fellow in training. He has authored over 350 national and international publications, delivered more than 500 presentations at national and international conferences, and contributed to more than 20 book chapters. Dr. Özdemir has also edited 10 books.

Contents

Preface

This book, titled *Asthma – Diagnosis, Management and Comorbidities*, includes nine chapters organized into five sections: "Introduction", "From Pathophysiology to Clinic", "Asthma in Allergy Clinics", "Difficulties to Manage Asthma", and "Differential Diagnosis".

Chapter 1 discusses the knowledge about asthma for general readers.

Chapter 2 begins by discussing airway remodeling, which plays a crucial role in asthma pathophysiology, and proceeds to explain how pulmonary fibrosis can develop in these patients and what should be done about it. It is a very interesting chapter.

Chapter 3 explains the distinction between primary and secondary immunodeficiencies, which play a crucial role in the diagnosis, treatment, and long-term care of asthma, as well as the importance of vaccinations for these patients and key considerations to be aware of.

Chapter 4 examines the relationship between asthma and primary ciliary dyskinesia in detail, beginning with its pathophysiology and proceeding to therapeutic approaches.

Chapter 5 deals with severe asthma, which is a real problem in clinical practice. This chapter discusses the phenotypes, endotypes, and their therapeutic responses and management in severe asthma.

Chapter 6 focuses on the relationship between pregnancy and asthma, including how to manage asthma during this period and the importance of asthma care.

Chapter 7 addresses Asthma-COPD Overlap, a topic that has recently gained renewed attention and is discussed in this chapter. The focus has been on the effect and role of sex in this overlap.

Chapters 8 and 9 will discuss the differential diagnosis of asthma in childhood and adulthood.

I would like to thank Publishing Process Manager Mirna Papuga and the entire IntechOpen staff for their assistance throughout the publication process. I would also like to thank my dear wife, Seval Hülya Özdemir, and my dear daughter, Berrin Nikame Özdemir, for their support during the preparation of this book.

Öner Özdemir MD
Division of Pediatric Allergy / Immunology,
Sakarya University Medical Faculty,
Research and Training Hospital,
Sakarya, Türkiye

Section 1

Introduction

Chapter 1

Introductory Chapter: Recent Developments in Diagnosis, Management, and Comorbidities of Asthma

Öner Özdemir

1. Introduction

Asthma is a chronic inflammatory pulmonary condition of the lower airways that affects your breathing and is characterized by typical symptoms of intermittent dyspnea, dry cough, and wheezing. Although the difficulties in the diagnosis of asthma in children still persist, it is easier through pulmonary function tests, as is known in adults. Although there have been no major innovations in its diagnosis in recent years [1–4], new biological agents have recently been developed and are frequently used in its treatment [5]. It is easier to recognize the comorbidities of asthma in our time, and there are innovations in the treatment approaches for these comorbidities.

This book aims to review recent advances in the diagnosis, treatment, and management of asthma and its comorbidities and to provide an update on current developments.

2. An overview of diagnosis of asthma

Guidelines for the diagnosis of asthma and new diagnostic advances in research in this field are very limited. The diagnosis is still mainly based on anamnesis, especially under the age of 5 years, and some known pulmonary function tests in adolescents and adults [1–4]. Chest CT has been partially and recently used in the diagnosis, although chest CT and functional lung imaging have recently been tried [3]. Again, the use of parameters other than NO in breath analysis for diagnostic and therapeutic purposes has started to increase [6]. Beyond diagnosing asthma, studies to determine asthma phenotypes and endotypes have come to the forefront in order to plan treatment [7, 8].

Recently, the differential diagnosis of asthma and its relationship with other diseases, such as chronic obstructive pulmonary disease (COPD), primary ciliary dyskinesia, and primary immunodeficiencies, have come to the forefront, and care plans are being developed for these diseases. In this book, we have chapters on these diseases, and the reader will be informed about these issues in detail.

3. Current treatment/management of asthma

Maintenance and Reliever Therapy (MART) has recently become very prominent in the treatment of asthma and is generally accepted among allergists worldwide [3]. The use of different biological agents, such as monoclonal antibodies (e.g., mepolizumab), in the treatment of asthma [5], especially in severe/resistant and uncontrolled types, has come to the forefront according to phenotype/endotypes [5, 9, 10]. Again, treatment and care plans are tried to be developed depending on the relationship or association with other comorbid diseases (COPD), primary ciliary dyskinesia, primary immunodeficiencies, etc.). Again, care and treatment plans, such as vaccination in asthmatic patients [11], coping with complications such as exacerbations during pregnancy, and development of pulmonary fibrosis, etc., are included in different chapters of this book and will definitely be useful to our readers.

4. The comorbidities of asthma

Asthma has many well-known comorbidities. Comorbidities are very important conditions for the diagnosis and treatment of asthma, and unless they are recognized or avoided, neither the diagnosis can be confirmed nor the treatment defined. These comorbidities include rhinitis, gastroesophageal reflux disease, vocal cord dysfunction, nasal polyposis, and bronchiectasis [12, 13]. It is important to note that asthma can also be comorbid with pulmonary fibrosis, COPD, primary ciliary dyskinesia, and primary/secondary ımmunodeficiencies [14, 15]. These issues are discussed in detail in our book and recent highlights are discussed.

5. Conclusion

I hope that the chapters in this book on the diagnosis and treatment of asthma and its comorbid disorders, written in the light of current literature, will change the diagnostic and therapeutic approaches of allergy and pulmonology specialists, and lead to a better and more accurate management of these diseases. I sincerely hope that this book, with its interesting chapters, will be useful to all physicians and other readers.

Author details

Öner Özdemir
Division of Pediatric Immunology and Allergic Diseases, Sakarya University Medical Faculty, Sakarya Training and Research Hospital, Sakarya, Türkiye

*Address all correspondence to: onerozdemir@sakarya.edu.tr

References

[1] Saxena S, Rosas-Salazar C. Diagnosing asthma in children. Respiratory Care. 2025;**70**(6):619-631. DOI: 10.1089/respcare.12543

[2] What is new in GINA 2025? Available from: https://ginasthma.org/gina-2025-slide-sets/ [Accessed: June 22, 2025]

[3] Lee C, Biederer J, Ohno Y, Seo JB, Parraga G, Levin DL, et al. International workshop for functional pulmonary imaging (IWPFI). Functional lung imaging using CT: An update. Radiology: Cardiothoracic Imaging. 2025;7(3):e240505. DOI: 10.1148/ryct.240505

[4] Gruffydd-Jones K. BTS/NICE/SIGN guideline for asthma 2024: Diagnosis, monitoring and chronic asthma management. How does this compare to GINA 2024? NPJ Primary Care Respiratory Medicine. 2025;**35**(1):22. DOI: 10.1038/s41533-025-00425-x

[5] Okwuofu EO, Chee Hui AY, Chee Woei JL, Stanslas J. The era of multiple biologics: Is combination and switching an option in the Management of Severe Asthma? Pulmonary Pharmacology & Therapeutics. 2025:102375. DOI: 10.1016/j.pupt.2025.102375

[6] Gagliani C, Brinkman P, Del Riccio M, Benfante A, Shahbazi Khamas S, Maitland-van der Zee AH, et al. Advances in exhaled breath condensate markers for severe asthma management: A systematic review. Expert Review of Respiratory Medicine. 30 Jun 2025:1-12. DOI: 10.1080/17476348.2025.2522743

[7] Chin-See-Chong TC, Kappen JH, Palmer E, Layhadi JA, Shamji MH, van der Valk JPM. Mechanisms and treatment of type 2 high and low asthma endotypes. Clinical and Experimental Allergy. 2025. DOI: 10.1111/cea.70084

[8] Ma J, Ma Q, Yang J, Liang P, Zhou J, Ma J, et al. The clinical and pathological histology efficacy of biological therapy for severe asthma with a phenotype of type 2 inflammation - Systematic review. Frontiers in Immunology. 2025;**16**:1531986. DOI: 10.3389/fimmu.2025.1531986

[9] Wirthgen E, Quickert S, Weitzel J, Salewski B, Ballmann M. Safety of biologics for the treatment of asthma in children and adolescents: A systematic review. European Respiratory Review. 2025;**34**(176):240269. DOI: 10.1183/16000617.0269-2024

[10] Xiao Q, Huang Y, Xue B, Wang M. The efficacy and safety of biologics for patients with severe asthma: An umbrella review of systematic reviews and meta-analyses. Frontiers in Medicine (Lausanne). 2025;**12**:1573596. DOI: 10.3389/fmed.2025.1573596

[11] Micheletto C, Aliberti S, Andreoni M, Blasi F, Di Marco F, Di Matteo R, et al. Vaccination strategies in respiratory diseases: Recommendation from AIPO-ITS/ETS, SIMIT, SIP/IRS, and SItI. Respiration. 2025:1-19. DOI: 10.1159/000544919

[12] Maselli DJ, Sherratt J, Adams SG. Comorbidities and multimorbidity in asthma. Current Opinion in Pulmonary Medicine. 2025;**31**(3):270-278. DOI: 10.1097/MCP.0000000000001162

[13] Bisaccioni C, Aun MV, Cajuela E, Kalil J, Agondi RC, Giavina-Bianchi P. Comorbidities in severe asthma: Frequency of rhinitis, nasal polyposis,

gastroesophageal reflux disease, vocal cord dysfunction and bronchiectasis. Clinics (São Paulo, Brazil). 2009;**64**(8):769-773. DOI: 10.1590/S1807-59322009000800010

[14] James AE, Abdalgani M, Khoury P, Freeman AF, Milner JD. T_H2-driven manifestations of inborn errors of immunity. The Journal of Allergy and Clinical Immunology. 2024;**154**(2):245-254. DOI: 10.1016/j.jaci.2024.05.007

[15] Vaseghi-Shanjani M, Samra S, Yousefi P, Biggs CM, Turvey SE. Primary atopic disorders: Inborn errors of immunity causing severe allergic disease. Current Opinion in Immunology. 2025;**94**:102538. DOI: 10.1016/j.coi.2025.102538

Section 2

From Pathophysiology to Clinic

Chapter 2

Airway Remodeling and Pulmonary Fibrosis in Asthma

Shima Rasouli

Abstract

Leukocyte invasion and tissue remodeling—including epithelial hyperplasia and collagen deposition—mark the common chronic inflammatory disease of the respiratory system. Clinically, it is characterized by airway inflammation, hyperresponsiveness, and airflow restriction, resulting in coughing, wheezing, and dyspnea. The pathogenesis of asthma involves a combination of immunological, environmental, and genetic factors. A significant component is airway remodeling, characterized by epithelial damage, smooth muscle hypertrophy, and fibrosis resulting from excessive extracellular matrix deposition. Linked to fibroblast-to-myofibroblast transition by TGF-β, fibrosis aggravates treatment resistance and severity of asthma—review of airway remodeling, lung fibrosis, mouse models, and asthma progression biomarkers.

Keywords: asthma, pulmonary fibrosis, airway remodeling, biomarkers, in vivo models

1. Introduction

Asthma is an inflammatory condition involving chronic lung involvement. Reversible obstruction, bronchial hyperresponsiveness (BHR), and persistent inflammation, brought on by the aberrant activity of Th2 lymphocytes, eosinophils, and mast cells, define it. Structural changes in the airways, sometimes referred to as airway remodeling, accompany the combined aberrant and exaggerated inflammatory activity of the immune system and cause life-threatening symptoms, including wheezing, coughing, and dyspnea [1–3].

Progressive changes in bronchial architecture brought about by chronic episodes of damage and repair define airway remodeling [4]. Epithelial tissue dysfunction, goblet cell hyperplasia, uncontrolled mucus production, and epithelial-mesenchymal transition (EMT)—which is started by the activation of fibroblasts and the beginning of fibrotic pathways—initiate the sum of these episodes of injury and repair [5]. Underneath the epithelium, these profibrotic pathways produce thickening of the basement membrane by aberrant production of growth factors including TGF-β, PDGF, and IL-13, resulting in the production and accumulation of collagen types I, III, and V and fibronectin along with excessive deposition of the extracellular matrix (ECM) [6].

An increase in muscle mass and aggravation in bronchoconstriction is linked to hyperplasia and hypertrophy of the airway smooth muscle layer [7]. Angiogenesis mediated by VEGF also results in vascular remodeling, increased blood supply, and, consequently, enhanced immune cell trafficking, which is linked to chronic inflammation [8]. Concurrently, an imbalance between matrix metalloproteinases (MMPs) and their inhibitors (TIMPs) aggravates the situation by increasing ECM turnover and extending structural changes. Particularly in severe asthma, the combination of these modifications reduces the bronchodilator response and its obstruction, contributing to airflow limitation [9]. Th2-mediated pathways are primarily responsible for the dysregulation of immune control in asthma, as they play a fundamental role in inflammation and remodeling [10]. First, Th2 cytokines, including IL-4, IL-5, and IL-13, stimulate pathways that lead to IgE generation and the recruitment of inflammatory eosinophils to the airways [11]. Second, Th2 chemokines, such as eotaxin, stimulate pathways leading to IgE generation and the recruitment of inflammatory eosinophils to the airways. Mast cells and eosinophils release cytotoxic granules and cytokines—IgE-mediated degranulation, histamine, and leukotrienes—which cause ongoing tissue damage, bronchospasm, and mucus secretion [12]. Generally, by inducing the dysregulated activity of myofibroblasts, the profibrotic activity of TGF-β is the primary axis of pathological extracellular matrix (ECM) protein accumulation in fibrosis of many organs, including the lung [13]. By stiffening the airway wall and thereby narrowing the lumen, these procedures lower pulmonary compliance [14].

Persistent immune signaling, epithelial damage, ECM accumulation, smooth muscle hypertrophy, mucosal gland hyperplasia, and neovascularization not only aggravate symptoms but also indicate a shift toward a more treatment-resistant disease phenotype [15, 16]. In more severe or chronically involved cases, all these fibrotic manifestations may extend into the lung parenchyma and contribute to progressive pulmonary fibrosis [17]. Otherwise, they may remain localized to the airways. Clinically, this shows signs of treatment-resistant asthma: persistent airflow restriction, more frequent exacerbations, and disturbed lung function despite best therapy [18].

The immunological and histological patterns in asthma pathology, which indicate fibrotic lesions, underscore the need to evaluate in vitro models and identify biomarkers as practical tools for tracking and detecting airway remodeling and fibrotic development. Type 2 inflammatory markers, including IL-13, periostin, FeNO, circulating ECM (e.g., MMPs, TIMPs), and epithelial damage, have so far given important new perspectives on the disease phenotype and response to treatment [19, 20]. Their inclusion into clinical practice could enable more exact and individualized treatments and early identification of patients at risk of irreversible damage [21].

This chapter attempts to give a summary of the processes behind airway changes causing fibrosis in asthma. Reviewing the cellular and molecular drivers of these structural changes, the experimental models used to investigate them, and the biomarkers that enable their detection, will help us to highlight present difficulties and future directions in the management of fibrotic asthma, thus bridging the gap between pathophysiological knowledge and clinical application.

2. Airway remodeling leading to pulmonary fibrosis in asthma

Airway structural changes in asthma are caused by a chronic, persistent, and maladaptive inflammatory response, leading to epithelial damage. Over time, these structural changes become persistent and stable, altering the bronchial wall and disrupting its functional integrity [1]. Etiologically, this accumulation of unresolved tissue repair results from repeated inflammatory episodes, often triggered by exposure to environmental irritants such as allergens, pollutants, and respiratory infections. In contrast to transient increases in respiratory responses, remodeling represents a permanent reorganization of airway structure resulting from chronic inflammation, which contributes to persistent airflow obstruction and a progressive decline in lung function, often in the form of pulmonary fibrosis [22]. Pulmonary fibrosis following remodeling in asthma occurs due to changes in various layers of the respiratory system's tissues.

At the epithelial interface, increased vulnerability of the pseudostratified columnar epithelium to stimuli occurs with the loss of tight junction proteins such as ZO-1 and occludin [23]. This disruption compromises the barrier function of this surface as part of the innate immune system, leading to increased epithelial permeability to allergens and microbes. Compensatory repair mechanisms are activated in a compensatory process, with actions including basal cell proliferation and aberrant differentiation, leading to goblet cell metaplasia via the Notch signaling pathway [24]. The latter contributes to obstruction and airflow limitation by overproducing MUC5AC and other gel-forming mucins, forming thick mucus plugs.

Subjacent to the epithelium, the lamina propria undergoes extensive remodeling characterized by the deposition of disorganized ECM components, including collagens I, III, and V. Activated fibroblasts and myofibroblasts—driven by profibrotic mediators such as transforming growth factor-beta 1 (TGF-β1)—are key contributors to this fibrotic response [25]. TGF-β1 induces fibroblast-to-myofibroblast transition (FMT) through canonical Smad2/3 signaling, along with non-canonical pathways such as PI3K/Akt and MAPK, promoting synthesis of ECM proteins and reinforcing tissue stiffness [26]. As a result, the reticular basement membrane (RBM) thickens, often exceeding 7–10 μm, a histological hallmark of chronic asthma [27].

ASM, as another major target in regeneration, not only increases in thickness through hyperplasia and hypertrophy but also undergoes proliferative and disabling changes of the muscles [28]. Firstly, PDGF and VEGF, as the central mitogenic stimulus involved in this layer, activate intracellular pathways including ERK1/2 and Akt [29]. These hypertrophic smooth muscle cells show increased contraction in response to cholinergic stimuli and decreased relaxation in response to β2 agonists, contributing to bronchial hyper-responsiveness and resistance to bronchodilators [30]. Secondly, since ASM is naturally rich in vascularity, it is a good target for angiogenesis of bronchial micro-vessels through the upregulation of VEGF and other proangiogenic mediators [31, 32]. Neovascularization, on the other hand, increases the density and permeability of newly formed, immature, and leaky vessels. Finally, ASM is rich in immune cells, including mast cells, lymphocytes, plasma cells, and macrophages, and this condition becomes more prone to further recruitment of leukocytes, resulting in increased airway wall edema during exacerbations, leading to chronic inflammation and further tissue remodeling. The condition is also exacerbated by remodeling of the airway neural elements, with increased sensory nerve fiber density and altered neuropeptide signaling (e.g., substance P, neurokinin A), thus enhancing bronchoconstriction and cough [33]. Meanwhile, enrichment of the peri-bronchial matrix with the matricellular proteins fibronectin, periostin, and tenascin-C acts as a positive feedback loop for further support of fibroblast activation and epithelial-mesenchymal interactions [34].

The combined effect of the structural changes mentioned is to form a narrowed and stiffened airway with reduced elasticity and impaired parenchymal connectivity. These changes perpetuate the chronic inflammatory state through persistent airway blockade, as well as by inducing a pro-inflammatory microenvironment [18]. Notably, these structural changes often persist even after the resolution of acute inflammation and are only marginally reversible with available anti-inflammatory therapies [35].

Thus, understanding the interconnected pattern of airway remodeling and the immunological signaling pathways involved is crucial for understanding the progressive nature of asthma and for developing treatments that go beyond symptomatic control. In particular, it has been shown that conventional corticosteroids effectively reduce airway inflammation but have limited efficacy in reversing the structural changes that have occurred. Therefore, targeted interventions with biologic drugs against key drivers of the pathophysiology of fibrosis in asthma (IL-13, IL-5, and TGF-β), or EMT and ECM modulators – to halt or at best reverse airway remodeling in severe asthma phenotypes – are under investigation [36, 37].

2.1 Role of chronic inflammation

In asthma, chronic inflammation perpetuates a vicious cycle of constant and abnormal damage and repair, altering the overall and cellular architecture of the airway over time. Unlike what happens in normal immune responses to immunogens, this constant local inflammation is driven by a complex collaboration of innate and adaptive immune cells including Th2 lymphocytes, eosinophils, basophils, and mast cells, neutrophils, and M2 macrophages, which individually and collectively generate and amplify profibrotic signals directly affecting the structure and function of airway tissue cells [2, 38].

Through their unique cytokines, IL-4, IL-5, and IL-13, Th2 cells are essential for coordinating and enhancing inflammatory and remodeling signaling pathways in allergic asthma (type I hypersensitivity) [10]. Particularly, IL-13 is dual; it not only causes goblet cell metaplasia and mucus hypersecretion in epithelial cells by activating STAT6, but also increases TGF-β1, hence fostering fibroblast-to-myofibroblast transition (FMT) [39]. Furthermore, encouraging the development and aggravation of the profibrotic milieu by inducing periostin from airway epithelial cells, IL-13 thus stimulates myofibroblast activity and ECM synthesis [34]. IL-4 and IL-13 both stimulate the activation of alternative macrophages and promote additional fibroblast proliferation through the IL-4Rα receptor.

The early phase of type I hypersensitivity results from the interaction between TH2 activation and the corresponding B lymphocytes producing IgE, which, upon subsequent exposure, binds to its receptor (FCεR) on the surface of basophils and mast cells, releasing inflammatory mediators (histamine, leukotrienes, prostaglandins, and cytokines) [40]. By generating IL-4, activated basophils help to differentiate α-SMA+ myofibroblasts and profibrotic M2 macrophages towards fibrosis and hence aggravate inflammatory conditions [41].

Especially in allergic-eosinophilic asthma, eosinophils are the characteristic effector cells in the late phase of type I hypersensitivity; they degranulate cytotoxic proteins such as basic master protein (MBP), eosinophil peroxidase (EPX), and eosinophil cationic protein (ECP), causing epithelial cell damage and barrier dysfunction. Apart from their damaging power, eosinophils also release TGF-β and FGF, which stimulate subepithelial fibroblasts and raise ECM deposition [11, 42, 43]. IL-5 and

GM-CSF guarantee continuous tissue damage and remodeling, therefore providing the feedback required for their long-term survival in inflamed tissues.

Alveolar macrophages in asthmatic airways simultaneously shift towards an M2 phenotype, characterized by elevated levels of TGF-β and PDGF, two key components that promote fibroblast proliferation and collagen production [44]. These macrophages also release acidic mammalian chitinase (AMCase) and breast regression protein-39/YKL-40 (chitinase 3-like 1), both of which increase fibroblast migration and ECM synthesis, and polarize more macrophages to the M2 phenotype, thereby deepening the fibrotic response [45].

In non-allergic eosinophilic asthma, the activation of group-2 innate lymphoid cells (ILC-2) triggered by alarmin (cytokines IL-22 and IL-33) produced IL-4, IL-5, and IL-13, respectively, thereby promoting Th2 differentiation, activation, and survival of eosinophils, and mucus secretion [46]. Furthermore, the synthesis of IL-5 and IL-13, as well as amphiregulin, by ILC-2 results in more eosinophils being recruited and their stimulation generating profibrotic cytokines (IL-13, TGF-β, and PDGF), hence increasing the fibroblast-to-myofibroblast transition [47].

Furthermore, in non-allergic, severe, corticosteroid-resistant neutrophilic asthma (where a Th17 axis generates IL-17, TNF-α, IFN-γ, and IL-6), most of the neutrophils are found at the site [48]. Tissue breakdown in the environment is caused in part by neutrophil degranulation (elastase, MMPs, etc.). However, these same neutrophils, provided by Th17, are a direct source of TGF-β, thereby augmenting the vicious cycle of repetitive damage and improper repair.

TGF-β is a master regulator of airway remodeling at the core of this inflammatory-fibrotic axis [49]. TGF-β initiates Smad2/3 phosphorylation upon binding to its receptor (TGFβRII), leading to nuclear translocation and transcription of profibrotic genes, such as COL1A1 and ACTA2. Activation of non-Smad-dependent pathways concurrently, including MAPK and PI3K/Akt, drives matrix synthesis and myofibroblast development [50]. Profibrotic inflammatory and anti-inflammatory cells, as well as cytokines, work together in a continuous cycle of immune activation and structural distortion, leading to increasing airway stiffness and narrowing. This progressively lowers lung compliance and airflow, ultimately producing ongoing airflow obstruction. This process is slow; hence, it usually remains unnoticed until significant functional impairment has occurred [51, 52]. Recent therapies have directly targeted these fibrotic pathways; agents such as dupilumab (blocking IL-4Rα) and pirfenidone (targeting TGF-β signaling) have the potential to disrupt this maladaptive remodeling process and change disease progression in patients with advanced asthma [53, 54]. This complex of causes of severe asthma is not responsive to conventional anti-inflammatory therapies.

2.2 Remodeling links asthma to pulmonary fibrosis

Remodeling in asthma is characterized by thickening of the smooth muscle around the airways, hyperplasia of mucous glands with a subsequent increase in mucus production, inflammatory damage to the epithelium, followed by increased accumulation of ECM under the epithelium as a repair response, and ultimately angiogenesis in the bronchi and bronchioles [55]. These events lead to relative narrowing and stiffness of the airways, but are usually controllable and even reversible with anti-inflammatory treatments (such as corticosteroids).

Chronic asthma in severe or incurable form, with repeated and intertwined episodes of inflammation and attempts to repair the resulting damage, often leads to pulmonary fibrosis. Here, the involvement of the lung parenchyma encompasses the subepithelial and interstitial layers, but it is localized, unlike the diffuse parenchymal fibrosis that occurs in the idiopathic form of pulmonary fibrosis. Remodeling culminates in tissue fibrosis, centered on the activity of profibrotic factors, the conversion of fibroblasts to myofibroblasts, and the extensive deposition of extracellular matrix (ECM), including collagen, fibronectin, and tenascin.

Activation of a network of signaling molecules centered on TGF-β binding to its receptor, both canonical and non-canonical pathways, results in increased transcription of profibrotic genes, including genes encoding α-SMA (a marker of myofibroblast differentiation) and various collagen isoforms (I, III, and V) to increase ECM [56]. Maintenance of the produced ECM is also exacerbated by TGF-β, which decreases and increases the expression of MMPs and TIMPs, respectively [57]. TGF-β, in the presence of IL-13 and other fibrogenic stimuli, stimulates resident fibroblasts in the airway wall to differentiate into contractile, ECM-producing myofibroblasts [58]. By exerting contractile force, α-SMA+ myofibroblasts stiffen the collagen-rich ECM beneath the epithelial layer and within the reticular basement membrane, thereby reducing lumen diameter and reducing flexibility, resulting in airway narrowing and decreased compliance [59]. This profibrotic matrix provides a rich environment for fibroblast self-activation and survival, and the true meaning of the positive feedback loop is an endless, permanent fibrotic cycle, accompanied by a corresponding permanent reduction in respiratory capacity and lung function.

It is of great importance to determine the prognosis of early fibrotic changes by biomarkers such as periostin, YKL-40, and collagen fragments (sputum or serum) of the fibrosis, and to identify patients at risk of irreversible fibrotic remodeling [60]. The development of targeted antifibrotic strategies, focusing on inhibiting TGF-β signaling with therapies such as pirfenidone and galonisertib, could focus on reducing the activity of stimulated fibroblasts or blocking immune activation mediated by inflammatory molecules such as TREM-1 [61, 62]. The latter option raises the question of the timing of the use of antifibrotic therapies, which are likely to be most effective only if initiated before fibrosis has developed, necessitating early diagnosis and targeted therapy based on the phase of the disease to preserve lung structure and function [63].

2.3 Factors influencing remodeling and fibrosis

The intricate interaction and interconnections among genetic vulnerability, epigenetic control, and environmental factors define the degree of airway remodeling and advancement of fibrosis in asthma [64]. Especially those encoding A disintegrin and metalloproteinase (ADAM33), TGF-β1, and IL-13, genetic predisposition is a significant determinant of the degree of vulnerability of an individual to airway structural changes arising from gene polymorphisms (factors that increase or decrease mRNA stability, increase or decrease transcription factor binding, RNA splicing alterations, overexpression, and gain-of-function) on inflammatory and fibrotic pathways [65]. Through the TGF-β and Wnt pathways, ADAM33 polymorphisms increase the expression of this membrane metalloproteinase in airway smooth muscle cells and fibroblasts, thereby stimulating the proliferation of these cells and causing adhesion and matrix interactions [66]. This accelerates remodeling in subepithelial fibrosis. Similarly, polymorphisms in TGF-β1 (e.g., rs1800470, also known as the +869 T/C variant) increase fibroblast activation, ECM protein synthesis, and airway wall thickening by increasing protein expression or its receptors, and amplifying signaling by upregulating profibrotic signaling protein Th2 cytokine genes may also undergo similar modifications, especially IL-4 and IL-13, which induce type 2 inflammation by several mechanisms including enhanced eosinophil recruitment, IgE generation, and epithelial-mesenchymal transition (EMT), thus accelerating fibrotic airway remodeling [10, 67]. Furthermore, linked to the control of TGF-β signaling, myofibroblast development, and inflammatory responses are epigenetic mechanisms involving changed expression of microRNAs, including miR-21, miR-155, and the let-7 family [68]. Moreover, DNA methylation changes in promoter regions of profibrotic genes (hypomethylation of TGF-β1, COL1A1, ADAM33, ACTA2, etc.) can enhance or repress gene transcription in response to environmental stimuli, thereby producing a dynamic regulatory layer that links chronic exposure to persistent airway structural changes [69].

Triggering genetic and epigenetic hazards are environmental elements, including chronic allergy exposure, air pollution, respiratory illnesses, and cigarette smoke [70]. Deeply penetrating the distal airways, fine air pollution particles (PM2.5, O_3, and NO_2) might induce hypomethylation of profibrotic genes [71]. Deeply penetrating the distal airways, fine air pollution particles (PM2.5, O_3, and NO_2) might induce hypomethylation of profibrotic genes [72–76]. The latter approach simultaneously lowers MMP activity and raises TIMP levels to help contribute more to ECM deposition [18]. Allergens (pollen, mites, animal dander, etc.) activate Th2 utilizing epithelial-derived alarmins such as IL-33, TSLP, and IL-25 and hypomethylation of Th2 genes (such as IL-4 and IL-13), therefore increasing ILC2s and prolonging eosinophilic inflammation [77]. By raising periostin and TGF-β, allergens also help fibroblasts to be activated and ECM to be formed [78]. Poor diet (such as folate and choline deficiency), chronic psychological stress (with altered methylation of the HPA axis), as well as elements such as heavy metals and occupational toxins are also known to be environmental factors that affect methylation changes and fibrosis [79]. Chronic viral infections (activation of IL-13, IL-33, methylation of immune genes, and increased fibrosis) are particularly relevant.

Clinically, this complicated relationship explains the observed variety in asthma phenotypes, notably severe and treatment-resistant forms that can lead to fibrotic obstruction [80]. Environmental triggers have synergistic effects with genetic polymorphisms and epigenetic alterations. Understanding the elements that cause fibrosis can help clarify risk factors, categorize asthma, predict prognosis, and identify potential sites for the application of pharmacological agents and optimal disease management in specific patients.

2.4 Impact of airway structural changes and fibrosis on asthma severity

The structural changes in the airways of asthmatic patients include thickening of the basement membrane leading to a concomitant decrease in airway elasticity and compliance, increased smooth muscle mass with increased severity of bronchospasm, hyperplasia of mucous glands leading to partial obstruction, persistent epithelial damage as a factor in the reduction of the defense barrier function and increased penetration of allergens and irritants, neovascularization with increased vascular permeability and chronic inflammation, and finally subepithelial fibrosis leading to increased airway resistance and a decrease in forced expiratory volume (FEV_1) [22, 55, 81–84]. This complex not only changes the anatomy but also fundamentally changes the behavior of the disease and the response to treatment [37]. As these processes of exaggerated destruction and remodeling progress, the nature of asthma changes from an episodic condition to a persistent and increasingly treatment-resistant state [85].

Although fibrosis in asthma is seen as subepithelial and is not as severe as diffuse fibrosis in ILD, after the progression of remodeling towards fibrosis in asthma, with increased airway wall thickness, decreased airway flexibility, and increased airflow resistance, it leads to increased symptom severity, decreased FEV_1, persistent obstruction, decreased response to bronchodilators, persistent dyspnea even without acute inflammation, and steroid deprivation (since fibrosis is also a non-inflammatory process), and sets the stage for refractory disease, especially in children, and severe asthma in adulthood due to early fibrosis [4, 86–88]. Thus, occasional breathing problems in patients gradually turn into persistent airflow limitation, and patients with long-term asthma often find it more difficult to control their symptoms over time, such that symptoms cannot be managed even with strong medications [89].

The main impact of these structural changes is on the response to treatment of the disease from a controllable state to a refractory form (refractory asthma) [90]. The reduced response to corticosteroids (the mainstay of asthma therapy) is due to the physical barrier of scar-like tissue formation to the drugs reaching their targets, and the lack of response to ICS in fibrosis is mainly because fibrosis is driven primarily by non-inflammatory pathways such as TGF-β, and is inherently insensitive to ICS [91]. In this regard, fibroblasts and myofibroblasts, the leaders in ECM synthesis, are very poorly responsive to glucocorticoids [92]. The thick and stiff wall loses the ability to mechanically respond to smooth muscle relaxation upon administration of bronchodilators (β_2-agonists) [93]. Biologic agents such as anti-IL-5 or anti-IL-13 may be only partially successful in controlling inflammation in the presence of advanced remodeling, but the obstruction remains persistent [94, 95].

Clinical studies have shown that patients with severe subepithelial fibrosis do not have a significant decrease in FEV_1 or the number of attacks despite the use of ICS/OCS, and despite conventional treatments, remodeling indices (such as wall thickness on CT or periostin levels) do not decrease in these individuals [96, 97]. For this reason, the focus of current research is on early detection of remodeling before fibrosis occurs through specific respiratory tests or biomarkers, rather than inflammation, and on the development of new therapies to correct and reverse these structural changes [98, 99].

2.5 Prospects for therapeutic intervention

New therapeutic strategies in line with molecular and cellular advances in the mechanisms of airway remodeling in asthma can pave the way for disease management beyond symptom relief, without focusing on inflammation and instead aiming to counteract tissue remodeling, fibrosis, and drug resistance, or even reverse airflow limitation in chronic asthma following fibrotic remodeling [100]. The most obvious agents are the direct antifibrotic therapies (inspired by IPF therapy), namely, pirfenidone and nintedanib for TGF-β and TNF-α inhibition, respectively, with proven antifibrotic effects and the inhibition of multiple tyrosine kinases (FGFR, PDGFR, and VEGFR) with promising effects in asthma [101–103].

Beyond anti-IgE and anti-IL-5 that target TSLP (tezepelumab) or TGF-β1 (e.g., fresolimumab) [104–107], biologic medicines targeting IL-13 are among the most exciting treatments. Anti-IL-13 lowers TGF-β1 and ECM [108, 109], thereby lowering remodeling. Targeting early upstream cytokines, so suppressing goblet cell metaplasia and mucus hypersecretion, and so indirectly lowering epithelial damage and downstream fibrotic responses, anti-TSLP targets fibrosis [110]. Though their use in asthma involves particular considerations and safeguards, anti-TGF-β1 targets the heart of fibrogenesis, even if their inhibitory effect provides major obstacles due to their broad-spectrum significance in immune control, tissue repair, and epithelial homeostasis [111]. Thus, more focused approaches, selectively inhibiting downstream signaling factors, emphasize the TGF-β/SMAD, Wnt/β-catenin (LGK974, ICG-001), and YAP/TAZ (Verteporfin) pathways, offering the potential to block profibrotic signaling and inhibit chronic inflammation-activated fibroplasia and fibroblast-to-myofibroblast differentiation without systemic immunosuppression [112]. Using histone deacetylase inhibitors to suppress the production of fibrogenic genes and DNA methyltransferase inhibitors to reduce methylation of the TGF-β or COL1A1 promoter, epigenetic treatments are being developed as a new method to treat resistant disorders [113]. Although the use of any of the above-listed medicines alone is insufficient, it is essential to include them in the therapy plan to control inflammation (e.g., with anti-IL-5), prevent remodeling and fibrosis (e.g., with anti-TGF-β), and potentially target epigenetics alongside them.

MMP-9/TIMP-1 balancers Batimastat, Marimastat by inhibiting MMPs (animal/in vitro trials) and TIMP-mimetics or siRNA to reduce TIMP-1 or regulate the balance to restore ECM homeostasis by correcting the imbalance between matrix degradation and accumulation [114–116]. Innovative molecular targets as a complement or alternative to existing treatments under investigation include balancing MMP-9 and TIMP-1 can be achieved using agents such as Batimastat and Marimastat (MMP inhibitors, tested in animal/in vitro studies) or TIMP-1 modulators, which aim to restore ECM homeostasis and reduce myofibroblast activation and persistence [117–120].

Personalized precision medicine will define airway remodeling therapy in the future. This includes identifying patients who are likely to require remodeling through biomarker panels (such as periostin, YKL-40, and TGF-β1 levels) combined with quantitative computed tomography (CT) imaging and high-resolution bronchial biopsies, thereby providing targeted biologics based on specific inflammatory or fibrotic endotypes and scheduling anti-fibrotic therapies before ECM deposition becomes permanent.

3. Murine models of airway remodeling and fibrosis

Mouse models are essential tools for studying asthma, providing a platform to investigate the mechanisms of airway remodeling and pulmonary fibrosis under controlled genetic and environmental conditions. While allowing for regulated genetic and environmental modification—benefits not possible in clinical research—these models closely reflect essential features of real disease [121]. Through specific sensitization and challenge strategies, mouse models facilitate the development of various asthma phenotypes, ranging from acute allergic inflammation to persistent structural alterations in the bronchial wall, including subepithelial fibrosis.

These models' practical relevance stems from their capacity to replicate the main characteristics of real asthma, including eosinophilic inflammation, enhanced airway responsiveness, mucus production, and airway wall thickening [121]. While genetically modified lines—such as transgenic or knockout mice—allow for the mechanistic study of individual signaling pathways involved in regeneration, including Th2-driven inflammation, TGF-β signaling, and epithelial-mesenchymal transition—the genetic homogeneity of inbred strains reduces inter-animal variability [122].

Within the framework of therapeutic development, mouse models offer significant benefits for assessing the efficacy of new drugs [121]. Their quick disease progression and short life cycle allow for fast assessment of treatments at several phases of the disease. Regarding the degree of regeneration, techniques such as high-resolution imaging, bronchial lavage (BAL), lung function tests (e.g., plethysmography), and histological assessment provide both quantitative and qualitative data [123]. Furthermore, applied to mouse tissues to expose cellular heterogeneity and signaling dynamics at high resolution are modern molecular techniques, including single-cell RNA sequencing, epigenetic profiling, and spatial transcriptomics [121]. Mouse systems are crucial for preclinical research, although no animal model can completely replicate the complex nature of human asthma. With humanized models, organoid cultures, and precise lung sections—which, when combined, help close the gap between basic research and clinical application—their value continues to grow [124]. Therapeutic targets and the temporal development of airway remodeling and fibrosis in asthma have been much clarified by insights from these developing platforms.

3.1 Asthma-fibrosis-related murine models

A wide range of murine models has been developed to investigate asthma-associated airway remodeling and fibrosis. These models differ in induction method, pathological features, and translational relevance. They include both allergen-driven asthma models that recapitulate airway remodeling and fibrosis-focused systems designed to unravel airway-centered fibrogenesis. **Table 1** summarizes the main models, their key advantages, and limitations. Together, they provide a versatile toolkit for dissecting fibrogenic pathways and testing potential therapeutics.

In addition to the models summarized in **Table 1**, other murine systems have also been developed. Allergen-based approaches such as fungal (*Aspergillus fumigatus*), cockroach, ragweed, and *Alternaria* largely resemble the house dust mite (HDM) paradigm, reproducing remodeling features but in more specific immunological contexts, for example, in steroid-resistant or fungal-sensitive asthma [145–147]. A different category encompasses advanced innovations, including humanized and double-humanized mice, multi-allergen or pollutant/virus exacerbation systems, asthma-to-fibrosis transition paradigms, CRISPR-based SNP models, and patient-derived xenografts (PDX) [148–153]. These platforms may offer greater translational fidelity than conventional models, but their complexity, cost, and lack of standardization have so far limited their widespread application. The specific scientific goals should ultimately inform model choice, balancing clinical relevance, experimental repeatability, and the remodeling qualities of interest.

3.2 Mechanistic insights from murine models of asthma-associated fibrosis

Murine models are becoming essential tools for elucidating the molecular and cellular processes underlying fibrosis in asthma and airway remodeling. Using these models, scientists have been able to precisely separate the dynamic interaction among cytokines, stromal cells, and signaling pathways that drive fibrotic remodeling both geographically and temporally. Among the primary signaling cascades linked, TGF-β remains the principal controller of fibrogenesis [154]. Utilizing both Smad2/3-dependent conventional signaling and non-canonical pathways, including MAPK, PI3K/Akt, and RhoA/ROCK, it stimulates fibroblast-to-myofibroblast

DOI: http://dx.doi.org/10.5772/intechopen.1011765

Model	Main induction	Key features	Molecules/pathways studied	Limitations	Relevance	Refs.
OVA	Sensitization + aerosol challenge	Eosinophilic inflammation, goblet cell metaplasia, subepithelial fibrosis	Th2 cytokines (IL-4, IL-5, IL-13), TGF-β	Artificial, poor translational value	Classical allergic asthma model	[125–130]
HDM	Chronic intranasal allergen	Smooth muscle hypertrophy, angiogenesis, long-term remodeling	TLR4 activation, epithelial alarmins (IL-25, IL-33, TSLP)	Variability, high cost	Closer to human asthma	[131–133]
Bleomycin	Intratracheal/ oropharyngeal instillation	Strong fibrosis, ECM deposition, honeycomb lesions	Pro-inflammatory cytokines (IL-1β, TNF-α), fibroblast activation	Acute injury, partial resolution	Gold-standard fibrosis model	[134–138]
CC10-TGFβ1	Inducible epithelial-specific overexpression	Subepithelial fibrosis, EMT	TGF-β/Smad signaling, EMT	Non-physiological induction	Mechanistic insights into TGF-β	[139]
CC10-IL-13	IL-13 overexpression	Alternative macrophage activation, fibrotic remodeling	IL-13/STAT6 pathway, periostin	Narrow scope	IL-13 pathway study	[140]
Terc−/−	Genetic knockout (telomerase-deficient)	Aging-related susceptibility to fibrosis	Telomere dysfunction	Limited scope	Models aging risk factors	[141]
AdTGFβ	Adenoviral TGF-β transduction	Strong peribronchial fibrosis	TGF-β axis	Acute, artificial	Airway-centric fibrosis	[142]
MMP9−/−, TIMP1−/−	Genetic knockout	Imbalance of ECM degradation vs. deposition	MMP/TIMP pathways	Not directly translational	ECM balance studies	[143, 144]

OVA, ovalbumin; HDM, house dust mite; Th2, T helper type 2; IL, interleukin; TSLP, thymic stromal lymphopoietin; AdTGFβ, adenoviral transforming growth factor-beta; CC10 (CCSP), club cell secretory protein; rtTA, reverse tetracycline-controlled transactivator; EMT, epithelial–mesenchymal transition; STAT6, signal transducer and activator of transcription 6; ECM, extracellular matrix; Muc5ac, mucin 5 AC; TLR4, toll-like receptor 4; TNF-α, tumor necrosis factor-alpha; MMP9, matrix metalloproteinase-9; TIMP1, tissue inhibitor of metalloproteinase-1; α-SMA, alpha-smooth muscle actin; PDGFRα, platelet-derived growth factor receptor-alpha; Terc−/−, telomerase RNA component knockout.

Table 1.
Comparative overview of murine models of asthma and pulmonary fibrosis.

transition (FMT), hence generating enhanced production of α-smooth muscle actin (α-SMA), collagen I, and fibronectin [155–158]. Crucially, mouse models have shown how TGF-β interacts with other signaling axes—most famously IL-13/STAT6—to generate a persistent fibrotic niche and enhance profibrotic gene expression [159]. IL-13 not only stimulates alternative macrophage activation but also causes periostin production by epithelial cells, hence improving ECM stiffness and myofibroblast activation [160, 161].

At the molecular level, epithelial-mesenchymal crosstalk is now a pillar of asthma-related fibrogenesis [162]. In mice, chronic allergen exposure causes epithelial production of alarmins, including IL-25, IL-33, and TSLP, which activate type 2 innate lymphoid cells (ILC2s), hence generating a Th2-dominant cytokine milieu [163]. These signals activate structural cell reprogramming in addition to immune cell invasion. Recent developments in single-cell RNA sequencing of mouse lungs have shown diverse fibroblast populations, including fractions with increased fibrogenic potential [164]. The growth of a "pathological fibroblast" subgroup defined by elevated expression of PDGFRα and profibrotic transcription factors, such as Sox9 and Twist1, during chronic remodeling is a particularly pertinent result [165, 166].

Additionally, mouse models are beneficial in clarifying the temporal development of fibrotic remodeling. Acute allergen challenge causes reversible epithelial hyperplasia, goblet cell metaplasia, and transient ECM deposition; prolonged exposure (6–12 weeks) causes irreversible structural changes, including airway smooth muscle (ASM) hypertrophy, subepithelial fibrosis, and basement membrane thickening [167]. Not only are mechanical cues from the ECM driving these persistent changes but also metabolic signals. Researchers have shown by in vivo imaging and lung stiffness mapping that higher matrix rigidity activates mechanosensitive pathways, including YAP/TAZ, hence increasing FMT and matrix deposition [168]. This mechanotransduction feedback loop implies that, even in the absence of continuous inflammation, fibrosis can turn self-perpetuating.

Murine studies also highlight another growing area of interest: the metabolic reprogramming of stromal cells during fibrotic remodeling. Supporting their biosynthetic and proliferative needs, myofibroblasts and stimulated epithelial cells exhibit a shift towards aerobic glycolysis—the Warburg effect [169]. This metabolic flexibility creates new options for therapeutic interventions targeting cellular bioenergetics in fibrotic asthma.

Crucially, these models have also specified important therapeutic windows for intervention. Early blocking of IL-13 has been demonstrated to prevent FMT and ECM buildup; yet, later-stage suppression of TGF-β or downstream effectors, including CTGF (connective tissue growth factor), can still somewhat reverse established fibrosis [170]. Murine systems do, however, also expose compensatory mechanisms that can complicate treatment plans. For example, genetic deletion of MMP9, supposed to lower matrix degradation, actually increases fibrosis because of altered ECM turnover and aberrant remodeling dynamics [171]. Likewise, cell-specific deletion models have defined the functions of airway epithelial cells, fibroblasts, and even ILC2s as essential mediators of fibrosis initiation and propagation, thus stressing the requirement of exact temporal and geographical targeting of antifibrotic treatments [172–174].

In terms of mechanistic discoveries in asthma-associated fibrosis, mouse models are somewhat effective overall. Under conditions that reflect key aspects of human disease, they enable a thorough dissection of molecular networks, the identification of new fibrogenic cell subsets, and the validation of potential therapeutic targets.

Particularly with the integration of lineage tracing, multi-omics profiling, and spatial transcriptomics, ongoing improvements to these models will help enhance our understanding of airway fibrogenesis and enable the development of more effective antifibrotic medicines.

3.3 Experimental utility and translational relevance of murine models in airway fibrosis research

For the mechanical dissection of airway remodeling and fibrosis in asthma, mouse models offer a unique and highly flexible platform. Their main advantage is their ability to enable high-resolution temporal and spatial control of disease induction, therefore enabling the gradual deconstruction of fibrotic cascades in ways both ethically and technically practical in human research. Researchers can investigate specific signaling nodes or cell populations in a context-dependent manner by using genetically engineered strains, thereby enabling a detailed understanding of cellular hierarchies and lineage dynamics during fibrotic progression.

These models have a significant benefit in being able to recreate intricate tissue architecture and extracellular matrix (ECM) changes seen in actual asthmatic lungs [175]. Validating these models as faithful approximations of human pathophysiology, subepithelial fibrosis, goblet cell metaplasia, smooth muscle hypertrophy, and accumulation of α-SMA+ myofibroblasts were all repeatably detected. Murine models reproduce the whole spectrum of cell-cell and cell-matrix interactions, including biomechanical feedback loops and paracrine signaling inside the fibrotic niche, unlike in vitro systems [168].

Particularly adapted for evaluating stage-specific therapies, the accelerated timeline of illness progression in mouse systems enables rapid longitudinal research. By use of modern imaging modalities, including micro-computed tomography (micro-CT), optical coherence tomography (OCT), and multiphoton microscopy, researchers may see dynamic structural changes and assess airway caliber, mucosal thickness, and tissue stiffness in vivo [176]. Complementing these instruments are invasive pulmonary function tests, such as flexiVent-based evaluations of airway resistance and elastance, which offer functional correlations to histological results [177].

Within the framework of drug development, mouse models serve as crucial intermediaries between in vitro screening and human trials. Evaluation of therapeutic efficacy in a controlled, disease-relevant environment has been made possible by their reactivity to biologicals aiming at profibrotic cytokines or mechanotransductive pathways. Post-treatment tissue studies, including immunohistochemistry, ECM profiling, and transcriptome analysis, also provide a mechanistic understanding of drug action, compensatory pathways, and possible biomarkers of response.

The usefulness of murine models has increased significantly with the advancement of genetic technologies. Conditional Cre-lox systems allow for temporal and cell-specific gene deletion, so allowing exact delineation of contributions from immunological, mesenchymal, and epithelial compartments [178]. Collagen I-GFP, α-SMA-RFP, and periostin-driven reporters, among other transgenic reporter strains, enable in vivo surveillance of fibrogenic activity and real-time evaluation of remodeling activities [179–181]. Increasingly utilized to validate treatment candidates, humanized mouse models—those incorporating elements of the human immune system or transgenic production of human cytokines—improve translational fidelity.

High-dimensional technology integration has recently improved the complexity of murine model analysis. These days, spatial transcriptomics, epigenomic profiling, and single-cell RNA sequencing (scRNA-seq) help to identify cellular heterogeneity and state transitions during remodeling [182]. Multiplexed imaging (e.g., CODEX) and mass cytometry (CyTOF) allow for deep phenotyping of immune cell populations and their interactions with stromal components [183]. These instruments offer unmatched clarity in delineating the cellular ecosystems in control of fibrogenesis.

Ultimately, high-throughput therapeutic screening is facilitated by the repeatability and scalability of mouse systems. Strong readouts matching human disease severity come from quantifiable endpoints like hydroxyproline content, airway thickness indices, and fibrotic gene signatures [184]. Many therapeutic approaches first found in mouse models—including metabolic inhibitors, epigenetic modulators, and integrin antagonists—have progressed to human trials, therefore supporting the predictive value of these systems for translational research (**Table 2**).

3.4 Structural and immunological limitations of murine models in fibrotic asthma

Murine models have several essential limitations that restrict their translational relevance to human asthma, even if they help to clarify basic processes of airway remodeling and fibrosis [121]. Anatomically, mouse lungs lack critical structural elements such as respiratory bronchioles and have a monopodial branching pattern different from that of human lungs [185]. These variations affect regional airflow dynamics and aerosol deposition, therefore changing the localization and degree of experimentally induced remodeling. Furthermore, in mice, the proportionately

Feature	Murine models	Human in vitro models (e.g., cell culture)	Large animal models (e.g., pigs, primates)
Similar to human pathology	Moderate to high (suitable for small airway remodeling)	Low (lack of 3D tissue architecture)	High (ideal for chronic changes and lung function studies)
Genetic control	Very high (transgenic, knockout, Cre-Lox)	Low (limited CRISPR use)	Very low
Time and cost	Short duration, low cost	Very low cost	Expensive and time-consuming
Imaging and longitudinal monitoring	High (micro-CT, in vivo imaging)	Low (needs organ-on-chip platforms)	High (MRI, CT, PET applicable)
Response to novel therapies	Reliable for early-stage testing	Useful for mechanistic insights	Appropriate for dose, pharmacokinetics, and safety testing
High-throughput screening feasibility	High	Very high	Very low
Distinct advantages	Detailed signaling analysis, localized remodeling	Precise cell-cell interaction analysis, direct use of human cells	Physiology closely mimics humans, long-term evaluation
Limitations	Physiological differences, limited for chronic modeling	Lacks full ECM and mechanical interactions	Ethical concerns, cost, and limited accessibility

Table 2.
Comparative evaluation of experimental models for asthma-associated pulmonary fibrosis.

bigger airway smooth muscle layers and different epithelial makeup may amplify or distort fibrotic reactions relative to human airways.

Significantly, interspecies variation exists in cytokine patterns, receptor expression, and effector cell function immunologically. For example, whilst Th cell polarization and innate lymphoid cell (ILC) subsets vary in frequency and activity, mouse eosinophils lack orthologs of important human granule proteins such as eosinophil-derived neurotoxin (EDN) [186]. Moreover, the relative predominance of Th2-driven responses in mouse models does not sufficiently reflect the spectrum of human asthma endotypes, especially Th1/Th17-skewed or non-type 2 (T2-low) asthma, which are often refractory to conventional therapies and underrepresented in preclinical pipelines [187].

One main restriction results from the nature of illness induction. Many mouse models depend on acute, high-dose allergen exposures (e.g., ovalbumin or HDM) or chemical agents (e.g., bleomycin), which generate exaggerated and temporally compressed fibrotic responses [188]. These systems frequently avoid the chronic, multivariate illness trajectory typical of human asthma, in which environmental exposures, viral infections, and host genetics interact over years. Moreover, damage caused by drugs like bleomycin or Ad-TGFβ reflects a type of direct cytotoxic insult that inadequately replicates the immune-mediated and repeated damage-repair cycles observed in asthma-associated airway remodeling [189].

Moreover, the interpretability of results is restricted by technical and methodological limitations. Because of their small lung size, mice are not suited for many non-invasive, longitudinal pulmonary tests applied in human research [190]. Most

Aspect	Strengths	Limitations
Anatomical relevance	Replicates key histopathological features, such as subepithelial fibrosis and myofibroblast accumulation.	Lacks true respiratory bronchioles, different airway branching, and thicker walls than human airways.
Immune system	Allows targeted manipulation of cytokines and immune cells to study immune-fibrotic interactions.	The immune system differs between humans and other species in cytokine profiles and immune cell composition.
Genetic manipulation	Availability of conditional knockouts and reporter strains for specific cell-type tracking.	Human gene promoters and regulatory sequences often behave differently in the murine context.
Disease induction	Models such as bleomycin and transgenic TGF-β enable focused studies of fibrosis.	Induction is often acute and non-physiologic compared to chronic, multifactorial asthma in humans.
Experimental control	Highly reproducible, with the ability to study temporal progression and intervention windows.	A compressed disease timeline may bypass the slow-developing remodeling seen in humans.
Drug testing	Efficient platform for preclinical therapeutic evaluation, including biologics and other therapeutic modalities.	Many agents effective in mice have failed in human trials due to interspecies differences.
Readout capability	Supports histological, molecular, and imaging analyses for detailed mapping of mechanisms.	Pulmonary function testing is invasive or terminal; mice cannot report subjective symptoms.
Translational relevance	Humanized and hybrid models increase relevance to human disease mechanisms.	Still limited in modeling non-Th2 asthma and inter-individual variability.

Table 3.
Advantages and limitations of murine models in airway remodeling and fibrosis research.

pulmonary function tests require terminal procedures, thereby restricting our understanding of disease development and treatment longevity. Central to asthma diagnosis, symptom evaluation is intrinsically complex in mouse systems and must rely on surrogate measures, including airway resistance or inflammatory cell counts, which do not always match patient-reported results [121].

Translationally, mouse models sometimes fall short in forecasting human treatment responses. Many biologics and small compounds have shown strong performance in preclinical asthma models, yet have produced negative findings in clinical studies [121]. This disparity reflects not only species-specific biology but also the simplistic and homogeneous character of mouse disease models compared to the genetic, environmental, and immunological diversity of human asthma populations.

These constraints taken together highlight the need to combine mouse results with organoids, human in vitro system data, and ex vivo tissue models [191]. Although mouse models are still indispensable for dissecting fundamental biological processes, their contribution to translational asthma research must be matched by more physiologically relevant and patient-specific platforms to ensure the development of successful, targeted treatments (**Table 3**).

4. Biomarkers of fibrosis formation in asthma

Biomarkers are objectively measurable indicators of biological or pathological processes, or of pharmacological responses to therapy. In asthma, particularly its fibrotic forms, biomarkers link clinical phenotypes with underlying molecular pathways. Unlike conventional diagnostic instruments, which primarily evaluate functional impairment, biomarkers offer a dynamic and molecular-level perspective on disease processes.

Early detection and stratification of patients based on risk for airway remodeling and fibrotic progression, real-time monitoring of disease activity and treatment responses, and long-term outcome prediction, including fixed airflow obstruction and therapy resistance, define three key roles for biomarkers in asthma-related fibrosis [98]. Through several biological matrices, including blood, bronchoalveolar lavage fluid (BALF), exhaled air, or tissue biopsies, these markers can be obtained, thereby facilitating both invasive and non-invasive evaluation approaches.

Crucially, since asthma spans a spectrum of inflammatory and structural endotypes, the discovery of fibrosis-specific biomarkers enables doctors and scientists to distinguish overlapping diseases and plan targeted treatments. Furthermore, in the era of precision medicine, biomarkers are becoming increasingly crucial for selecting suitable biologic treatments and for developing new antifibrotic drugs aimed at halting or slowing the structural degradation of the airways. Thus, emphasizing the need to characterize and monitor fibrotic remodeling as a unique and clinically relevant process, biomarker research is becoming a pillar of translational efforts to redefine asthma beyond inflammation. To provide a structured overview of these diverse biomarker categories and avoid redundancy, the main indicators discussed in subsequent sections are integrated into a comprehensive summary table (**Table 4**), highlighting their biological roles, clinical significance, and limitations.

Among the most intriguing opportunities in asthma research is the inclusion of biomarkers into precision medicine. Targeting therapies depending on the unique traits of every patient—including genetic, molecular, and phenotypic

Biomarker domain	Biomarker/molecule	Role in remodeling & fibrosis	Clinical/translational relevance	Limitations	Refs
Indicators of airway structural alterations	Collagen I, III, V; fibronectin; laminin	ECM deposition, basement membrane thickening	Histology, BALF/serum assays	Not asthma-specific	[192]
	MMP-2, MMP-9, TIMP-1	ECM degradation vs. inhibition	BALF/blood readouts; MMP/TIMP ratio may flag patients less responsive to corticosteroids	Variable, inconsistent	[193, 194]
	TGF-β1	Central profibrotic mediator; EMT, FMT, ECM synthesis	Measured in serum and BALF; biomarker and therapeutic target (resistance to conventional therapy in candidates for anti-TGF-β drugs)	Pleiotropic, context-dependent	[107, 195]
Immunoinflammatory signatures as predictors	IL-4, IL-5, IL-13	Th2 inflammation, eosinophilia, profibrotic signaling; periostin induction	Biologics (dupilumab, mepolizumab)	Only T2-high	[196, 197]
	Periostin	IL-13/TGF-β-driven ECM stiffness	Detected in serum and BALF; candidate non-invasive biomarker; elevated in poor response to anti-IL-13 biologics	Non-specific	[198, 199]
	Eosinophil counts	Th2 inflammation, TGF-β/IL-13-mediated fibrosis	Simple, accessible	Poor in T2-low asthma	[200, 201]
Circulating and tissue-derived biomarkers	YKL-40, AMCase (serum and BALF)	ECM turnover, linked to remodeling severity and fibrosis	Accessible biomarker across matrices (BALF and tissue), elevated YKL-40 under therapy may signal treatment resistance	Not disease-specific, exploratory; limited validation	[202–205]
	Fibulin-1	ECM glycoprotein; airway stiffness; TGF-β pathway	Serum biomarker	Limited validation	[206, 207]
	EBC/VOCs	Volatile organic compound signatures	Non-invasive, exploratory	Poor reproducibility	[208–210]
Genomic and epigenomic	IL-13 SNPs, TGF-β variants	Genetic susceptibility	Risk profiling	Low predictive power	[211–213]
	DNA methylation, Histone modifications	Epigenetic regulation	Omics biomarker discovery	No standardized assays	[214]

Biomarker domain	Biomarker/ molecule	Role in remodeling & fibrosis	Clinical/translational relevance	Limitations	Refs
Biomarker-driven stratification for therapy	TSLP, IL-25, IL-33, Muc5ac	Alarmin release, mucus metaplasia; drug targets	Biologics (e.g., tezepelumab); patient stratification	Mostly preclinical	[215–217]
	Proteomics and metabolomics	Integrated biomarker panels, systemic signatures	Precision stratification	Expensive, non-standardized	[218, 219]

Abbreviations: BALF, bronchoalveolar lavage fluid; ECM, extracellular matrix; MMP, matrix metalloproteinase; TIMP, tissue inhibitor of metalloproteinases; TGF-β, transforming growth factor beta; EMT, epithelial–mesenchymal transition; FMT, fibroblast–myofibroblast transition; IL, interleukin; SNP, single nucleotide polymorphism; DNA, deoxyribonucleic acid; TSLP, thymic stromal lymphopoietin; Muc5ac, mucin 5 subtype AC; EBC, exhaled breath condensate; VOCs, volatile organic compounds.

Table 4.
Representative biomarkers of airway remodeling and fibrosis in asthma: pathophysiological roles and translational relevance.

information—precision medicine seeks. This method primarily relies on biomarkers, as they provide the molecular insights necessary to select the most effective therapy plans.

Patients with particular fibrotic pathways can be identified using biomarkers, which allows focused treatments addressing the fundamental causes of fibrosis. For patients with high TGF-β levels, for instance, anti-TGF-β treatments—which block signals encouraging fibrosis—could be customized [220]. Likewise, anti-IL-13 treatments may be applied to patients with high levels of periostin, a marker of Th2-driven inflammation and remodeling [221].

Furthermore, enabling more tailored monitoring of therapy response will be the creation of patient-specific biomarker profiles. Through constant surveillance of relevant biomarkers, clinicians can adjust therapy instantly to maximize efficacy and minimize adverse effects. Patients whose fibrosis biomarkers remain high despite treatment, for example, may be driven to different medications or pursue more aggressive management schemes.

Eventually, precision medicine might lead to the development of biomarker-guided clinical studies, in which case-specific biomarkers indicate eligibility for participation in specific therapeutic procedures. This will guarantee that the correct treatments are tested in the appropriate patient populations as well as increase the efficiency of clinical studies.

5. Conclusion and future directions

Asthma is a diverse chronic condition in which ongoing inflammation can lead to structural changes in the airways, sometimes referred to as airway remodeling. This process may progress to pulmonary fibrosis in advanced or severe cases, leading to treatment resistance and irreversible airflow restriction. Emphasizing the interaction between immunological and fibrotic pathways, particularly the roles of TGF-β, IL-13, and MMPs in promoting extracellular matrix deposition and scarring, this chapter examines the fundamental processes of fibrotic remodeling in asthma.

Though its constraints—especially in simulating human illness heterogeneity—necessitate the adoption of more physiologically relevant systems, such as humanized mice or airway organoids, mouse models have been indispensable in clarifying these pathways. New opportunities for understanding the complex cellular connections involved in fibrosis arise from technological advancements such as single-cell profiling and high-resolution imaging.

This chapter primarily focused on identifying biomarkers indicative of fibrosis development in asthma. These include molecular markers found in blood, tissue, and exhaled breath, which would enable early detection, disease monitoring, and patient stratification. Although clinical translation and validation still present challenges, the combination of genetic, epigenetic, and multi-omics data has expanded the prospect for robust, clinically relevant biomarkers.

Though much has been accomplished, various obstacles prevent the creation of efficient antifibrotic treatments for asthma. Among these are a lack of knowledge about the multiple processes that cause fibrosis, inadequate sensitive and specific diagnostic methods, and underrepresentation of non-type two asthma phenotypes in preclinical studies. Furthermore, many of the current treatments primarily target upstream inflammation without directly addressing fibrogenesis.

Essentially, as we advance, a systems biology approach will be employed, including predictive modeling, precision medicine concepts, and multi-omics technology. Stratifying patients based on their genetic profiles can help, especially in those who are at risk for fibrotic development, to provide more tailored treatments. Dependent on the development of reliable, non-invasive biomarkers and enhancement of experimental models, improving diagnosis accuracy and therapy results will rely mainly on each other.

From generic treatment paradigms to targeted, mechanism-based care that addresses both inflammatory and fibrotic components of the disease, transforming the management of fibrotic asthma requires a multidisciplinary, tailored approach.

Author details

Shima Rasouli
Department of Immunology and Microbiology, TeMS.C., Islamic Azad University, Tehran, Iran

*Address all correspondence to: sh.rasouli.1984@gmail.com

References

[1] Holgate ST. Pathogenesis of asthma. Clinical and Experimental Allergy. 2008;**38**(6):872-897

[2] Lambrecht BN, Hammad H. The immunology of asthma. Nature Immunology. 2015;**16**(1):45-56

[3] Elias JA, Lee CG, Zheng T, Ma B, Homer RJ, Zhu Z. New insights into the pathogenesis of asthma. The Journal of Clinical Investigation. 2003;**111**(3):291-297

[4] Bergeron C, Boulet LP. Structural changes in airway diseases: Characteristics, mechanisms, consequences, and pharmacologic modulation. Chest. 2006;**129**(4):1068-1087

[5] Bousquet J, Jeffery PK, Busse WW, Johnson M, Vignola AM. Asthma. From bronchoconstriction to airways inflammation and remodeling. American Journal of Respiratory and Critical Care Medicine. 2000;**161**(5):1720-1745

[6] Al-Muhsen S, Johnson JR, Hamid Q. Remodeling in asthma. The Journal of Allergy and Clinical Immunology. 2011;**128**(3):451-462; quiz 63-4

[7] Johnson PR. Role of human airway smooth muscle in altered extracellular matrix production in asthma. Clinical and Experimental Pharmacology & Physiology. 2001;**28**(3):233-236

[8] Lee CG, Link H, Baluk P, Homer RJ, Chapoval S, Bhandari V, et al. Vascular endothelial growth factor (VEGF) induces remodeling and enhances TH2-mediated sensitization and inflammation in the lung. Nature Medicine. 2004;**10**(10):1095-1103

[9] Lagente V, Manoury B, Nénan S, Le Quément C, Martin-Chouly C, Boichot E. Role of matrix metalloproteinases in the development of airway inflammation and remodeling. Brazilian Journal of Medical and Biological Research. 2005;**38**(10):1521-1530

[10] Wills-Karp M, Luyimbazi J, Xu X, Schofield B, Neben TY, Karp CL, et al. Interleukin-13: Central mediator of allergic asthma. Science. 1998;**282**(5397):2258-2261

[11] Gleich GJ. Mechanisms of eosinophil-associated inflammation. The Journal of Allergy and Clinical Immunology. 2000;**105**(4):651-663

[12] Robinson DS. The role of the mast cell in asthma: Induction of airway hyperresponsiveness by interaction with smooth muscle? The Journal of Allergy and Clinical Immunology. 2004;**114**(1):58-65

[13] Holgate ST. Airway inflammation and remodeling in asthma: Current concepts. Molecular Biotechnology. 2002;**22**(2):179-189

[14] Wynn TA. Cellular and molecular mechanisms of fibrosis. The Journal of Pathology. 2008;**214**(2):199-210

[15] Ojiaku CA, Yoo EJ, Panettieri RA Jr. Transforming growth factor β1 function in airway remodeling and hyperresponsiveness. The missing link? American Journal of Respiratory Cell and Molecular Biology. 2017;**56**(4):432-442

[16] Postma DS, Timens W. Remodeling in asthma and chronic obstructive pulmonary disease. Proceedings

of the American Thoracic Society. 2006;**3**(5):434-439

[17] James AL, Wenzel S. Clinical relevance of airway remodelling in airway diseases. The European Respiratory Journal. 2007;**30**(1):134-155

[18] Vignola AM, Mirabella F, Costanzo G, Di Giorgi R, Gjomarkaj M, Bellia V, et al. Airway remodeling in asthma. Chest. 2003;**123**(3 Suppl):417s-422s

[19] Konradsen JR, Skantz E, Nordlund B, Lidegran M, James A, Ono J, et al. Predicting asthma morbidity in children using proposed markers of Th2-type inflammation. Pediatric Allergy and Immunology. 2015;**26**(8):772-779

[20] Robroeks CM, van de Kant KD, Jöbsis Q, Hendriks HJ, van Gent R, Wouters EF, et al. Exhaled nitric oxide and biomarkers in exhaled breath condensate indicate the presence, severity and control of childhood asthma. Clinical and Experimental Allergy. 2007;**37**(9):1303-1311

[21] Loza MJ, Djukanovic R, Chung KF, Horowitz D, Ma K, Branigan P, et al. Validated and longitudinally stable asthma phenotypes based on cluster analysis of the ADEPT study. Respiratory Research. 2016;**17**(1):165

[22] Jeffery PK. Remodeling and inflammation of bronchi in asthma and chronic obstructive pulmonary disease. Proceedings of the American Thoracic Society. 2004;**1**(3):176-183

[23] Xiao C, Puddicombe SM, Field S, Haywood J, Broughton-Head V, Puxeddu I, et al. Defective epithelial barrier function in asthma. The Journal of Allergy and Clinical Immunology. 2011;**128**(3):549-556.e1-12

[24] Danahay H, Pessotti AD, Coote J, Montgomery BE, Xia D, Wilson A, et al. Notch2 is required for inflammatory cytokine-driven goblet cell metaplasia in the lung. Cell Reports. 2015;**10**(2):239-252

[25] Redington AE. Airway fibrosis in asthma: Mechanisms, consequences, and potential for therapeutic intervention. Monaldi Archives for Chest Disease. 2000;**55**(4):317-323

[26] Gu L, Zhu YJ, Yang X, Guo ZJ, Xu WB, Tian XL. Effect of TGF-beta/Smad signaling pathway on lung myofibroblast differentiation. Acta Pharmacologica Sinica. 2007;**28**(3):382-391

[27] Roche WR, Beasley R, Williams JH, Holgate ST. Subepithelial fibrosis in the bronchi of asthmatics. Lancet. 1989;**1**(8637):520-524

[28] James A, Mauad T, Abramson M, Green F. Airway smooth muscle hypertrophy and hyperplasia in asthma. American Journal of Respiratory and Critical Care Medicine. 2012;**186**(6):568; author reply 9

[29] Hirst SJ, Martin JG, Bonacci JV, Chan V, Fixman ED, Hamid QA, et al. Proliferative aspects of airway smooth muscle. The Journal of Allergy and Clinical Immunology. 2004;**114**(2 Suppl):S2-S17

[30] Johnson PR, Roth M, Tamm M, Hughes M, Ge Q, King G, et al. Airway smooth muscle cell proliferation is increased in asthma. American Journal of Respiratory and Critical Care Medicine. 2001;**164**(3):474-477

[31] Salvato G. Quantitative and morphological analysis of the vascular bed in bronchial biopsy specimens from asthmatic and non-asthmatic subjects. Thorax. 2001;**56**(12):902-906

[32] Hoshino M, Takahashi M, Aoike N. Expression of vascular endothelial growth factor, basic fibroblast growth factor, and angiogenin immunoreactivity in asthmatic airways and its relationship to angiogenesis. The Journal of Allergy and Clinical Immunology. 2001;**107**(2):295-301

[33] Li M, Shang YX, Wei B, Yang YG. The effect of substance P on asthmatic rat airway smooth muscle cell proliferation, migration, and cytoplasmic calcium concentration in vitro. Journal of Inflammation (Lond). 2011;**8**(1):18

[34] Takayama G, Arima K, Kanaji T, Toda S, Tanaka H, Shoji S, et al. Periostin: A novel component of subepithelial fibrosis of bronchial asthma downstream of IL-4 and IL-13 signals. The Journal of Allergy and Clinical Immunology. 2006;**118**(1):98-104

[35] Boulet LP. Airway remodeling in asthma: Update on mechanisms and therapeutic approaches. Current Opinion in Pulmonary Medicine. 2018;**24**(1):56-62

[36] Olin JT, Wechsler ME. Asthma: Pathogenesis and novel drugs for treatment. BMJ. 2014;**349**:g5517

[37] Fahy JV. Type 2 inflammation in asthma--present in most, absent in many. Nature Reviews. Immunology. 2015;**15**(1):57-65

[38] Holgate ST. Innate and adaptive immune responses in asthma. Nature Medicine. 2012;**18**(5):673-683

[39] Kuperman DA, Huang X, Koth LL, Chang GH, Dolganov GM, Zhu Z, et al. Direct effects of interleukin-13 on epithelial cells cause airway hyperreactivity and mucus overproduction in asthma. Nature Medicine. 2002;**8**(8):885-889

[40] Miyake K, Ito J, Karasuyama H. Role of basophils in a broad spectrum of disorders. Frontiers in Immunology. 2022;**13**:902494

[41] Leask A. Getting to the heart of the matter: New insights into cardiac fibrosis. Circulation Research. 2015;**116**(7):1269-1276

[42] Kay AB. The role of eosinophils in the pathogenesis of asthma. Trends in Molecular Medicine. 2005;**11**(4):148-152

[43] Flood-Page PT, Menzies-Gow AN, Kay AB, Robinson DS. Eosinophil's role remains uncertain as anti-interleukin-5 only partially depletes numbers in asthmatic airway. American Journal of Respiratory and Critical Care Medicine. 2003;**167**(2):199-204

[44] Robbe P, Draijer C, Borg TR, Luinge M, Timens W, Wouters IM, et al. Distinct macrophage phenotypes in allergic and nonallergic lung inflammation. American Journal of Physiology. Lung Cellular and Molecular Physiology. 2015;**308**(4):L358-L367

[45] Lee CG, Da Silva CA, Dela Cruz CS, Ahangari F, Ma B, Kang MJ, et al. Role of chitin and chitinase/chitinase-like proteins in inflammation, tissue remodeling, and injury. Annual Review of Physiology. 2011;**73**:479-501

[46] Wirtz S, Schulz-Kuhnt A, Neurath MF, Atreya I. Functional contribution and targeted migration of group-2 innate lymphoid cells in inflammatory lung diseases: Being at the right place at the right time. Frontiers in Immunology. 2021;**12**:688879

[47] Mikami Y, Takada Y, Hagihara Y, Kanai T. Innate lymphoid cells in organ fibrosis. Cytokine & Growth Factor Reviews. 2018;**42**:27-36

[48] Habib N, Pasha MA, Tang DD. Current understanding of asthma pathogenesis and biomarkers. Cells. 2022;**11**(17):2764

[49] Derynck R, Zhang YE. Smad-dependent and Smad-independent pathways in TGF-beta family signalling. Nature. 2003;**425**(6958):577-584

[50] Willis BC, Borok Z. TGF-beta-induced EMT: Mechanisms and implications for fibrotic lung disease. American Journal of Physiology. Lung Cellular and Molecular Physiology. 2007;**293**(3):L525-L534

[51] Elias JA, Zhu Z, Chupp G, Homer RJ. Airway remodeling in asthma. The Journal of Clinical Investigation. 1999;**104**(8):1001-1006

[52] Tashkin DP, Wechsler ME. Role of eosinophils in airway inflammation of chronic obstructive pulmonary disease. International Journal of Chronic Obstructive Pulmonary Disease. 2018;**13**:335-349

[53] Noble PW, Albera C, Bradford WZ, Costabel U, Glassberg MK, Kardatzke D, et al. Pirfenidone in patients with idiopathic pulmonary fibrosis (CAPACITY): Two randomised trials. Lancet. 2011;**377**(9779):1760-1769

[54] Castro M, Corren J, Pavord ID, Maspero J, Wenzel S, Rabe KF, et al. Dupilumab efficacy and safety in moderate-to-severe uncontrolled asthma. The New England Journal of Medicine. 2018;**378**(26):2486-2496

[55] Hough KP, Curtiss ML, Blain TJ, Liu RM, Trevor J, Deshane JS, et al. Airway remodeling in asthma. Front Med (Lausanne). 2020;7:191

[56] Meng XM, Nikolic-Paterson DJ, Lan HY. TGF-β: The master regulator of fibrosis. Nature Reviews. Nephrology. 2016;**12**(6):325-338

[57] Frangogiannis N. Transforming growth factor-β in tissue fibrosis. The Journal of Experimental Medicine. 2020;**217**(3):e20190103

[58] Hinz B. Formation and function of the myofibroblast during tissue repair. The Journal of Investigative Dermatology. 2007;**127**(3):526-537

[59] Vallée A, Lecarpentier Y. TGF-β in fibrosis by acting as a conductor for contractile properties of myofibroblasts. Cell & Bioscience. 2019;**9**:98

[60] Korthagen NM, van Moorsel CH, Barlo NP, Ruven HJ, Kruit A, Heron M, et al. Serum and BALF YKL-40 levels are predictors of survival in idiopathic pulmonary fibrosis. Respiratory Medicine. 2011;**105**(1):106-113

[61] Giarratana AO, Prendergast CM, Salvatore MM, Capaccione KM. TGF-β signaling: Critical nexus of fibrogenesis and cancer. Journal of Translational Medicine. 2024;**22**(1):594

[62] Jing H, Gao Y, Jing L, Yang H, Liu S. Recent advances in therapeutic use of transforming growth factor-beta inhibitors in cancer and fibrosis. Frontiers in Oncology. 2025;**15**:1489701

[63] Raghu G, Rochwerg B, Zhang Y, Garcia CA, Azuma A, Behr J, et al. An official ATS/ERS/JRS/ALAT clinical practice guideline: Treatment of idiopathic pulmonary fibrosis. An update of the 2011 clinical practice guideline. American Journal of Respiratory and Critical Care Medicine. 2015;**192**(2):e3-e19

[64] Holgate ST. Epithelium dysfunction in asthma. The Journal of Allergy and Clinical Immunology. 2007;**120**(6):1233-1244; quiz 45-6

[65] Van Eerdewegh P, Little RD, Dupuis J, Del Mastro RG, Falls K, Simon J, et al. Association of the ADAM33 gene with asthma and bronchial hyperresponsiveness. Nature. 2002;**418**(6896):426-430

[66] Lee JY, Park SW, Chang HK, Kim HY, Rhim T, Lee JH, et al. A disintegrin and metalloproteinase 33 protein in patients with asthma: Relevance to airflow limitation. American Journal of Respiratory and Critical Care Medicine. 2006;**173**(7):729-735

[67] Grainger DJ, Heathcote K, Chiano M, Snieder H, Kemp PR, Metcalfe JC, et al. Genetic control of the circulating concentration of transforming growth factor type beta1. Human Molecular Genetics. 1999;**8**(1):93-97

[68] Lu TX, Rothenberg ME. MicroRNA. The Journal of Allergy and Clinical Immunology. 2018;**141**(4):1202-1207

[69] Yang IV, Schwartz DA. Epigenetic control of gene expression in the lung. American Journal of Respiratory and Critical Care Medicine. 2011;**183**(10):1295-1301

[70] Peden DB, Bush RK. Advances in environmental and occupational disorders 2006. The Journal of Allergy and Clinical Immunology. 2007;**119**(5):1127-1132

[71] Liu K, Hua S, Song L. PM2.5 exposure and asthma development: The key role of oxidative stress. Oxidative Medicine and Cellular Longevity. 2022;**2022**:3618806

[72] Zong D, Liu X, Li J, Ouyang R, Chen P. The role of cigarette smoke-induced epigenetic alterations in inflammation. Epigenetics & Chromatin. 2019;**12**(1):65

[73] Anderson R, Theron AJ, Richards GA, Myer MS, van Rensburg AJ. Passive smoking by humans sensitizes circulating neutrophils. The American Review of Respiratory Disease. 1991;**144**(3 Pt 1):570-574

[74] Overbeek SA, Braber S, Henricks PA, Kleinjan M, Kamp VM, Georgiou NA, et al. Cigarette smoke induces β2-integrin-dependent neutrophil migration across human endothelium. Respiratory Research. 2011;**12**(1):75

[75] Birru RL, Di YP. Pathogenic mechanism of second hand smoke induced inflammation and COPD. Frontiers in Physiology. 2012;**3**:348

[76] Woodruff PG, Ellwanger A, Solon M, Cambier CJ, Pinkerton KE, Koth LL. Alveolar macrophage recruitment and activation by chronic second hand smoke exposure in mice. COPD. 2009;**6**(2):86-94

[77] Licona-Limón P, Kim LK, Palm NW, Flavell RA. TH2, allergy and group 2 innate lymphoid cells. Nature Immunology. 2013;**14**(6):536-542

[78] Woodruff PG, Modrek B, Choy DF, Jia G, Abbas AR, Ellwanger A, et al. T-helper type 2-driven inflammation defines major subphenotypes of asthma. American Journal of Respiratory and Critical Care Medicine. 2009;**180**(5):388-395

[79] Miller RL, Peden DB. Environmental effects on immune responses in patients with atopy and asthma. The Journal of Allergy and Clinical Immunology. 2014;**134**(5):1001-1008

[80] Wenzel SE. Asthma phenotypes: The evolution from clinical to molecular approaches. Nature Medicine. 2012;**18**(5):716-725

[81] James AL, Donovan GM, Green FHY, Mauad T, Abramson MJ, Cairncross A, et al. Heterogeneity of airway smooth muscle remodeling in asthma. American Journal of Respiratory and Critical Care Medicine. 2023;**207**(4):452-460

[82] Bergeron C, Tulic MK, Hamid Q. Airway remodelling in asthma: From benchside to clinical practice. Canadian Respiratory Journal. 2010;**17**(4):e85-e93

[83] Ogulur I, Pat Y, Yazici D, Ardicli S, Ardicli O, Mitamura Y, et al. Epithelial barrier dysfunction, type 2 immune response, and the development of chronic inflammatory diseases. Current Opinion in Immunology. 2024;**91**:102493

[84] Pałgan K, Bartuzi Z. Angiogenesis in bronchial asthma. International Journal of Immunopathology and Pharmacology. 2015;**28**(3):415-420

[85] Busse WW, Lemanske RF Jr. Asthma. The New England Journal of Medicine. 2001;**344**(5):350-362

[86] Di Cicco M, Ghezzi M, Kantar A, Song W-J, Bush A, Peroni D, et al. Pediatric obesity and severe asthma: Targeting pathways driving inflammation. Pharmacological Research. 2023;**188**:106658

[87] Wenzel S. Severe asthma: From characteristics to phenotypes to endotypes. Clinical and Experimental Allergy. 2012;**42**(5):650-658

[88] Fang L, Roth M. Airway Wall remodeling in childhood asthma-a personalized perspective from cell type-specific biology. J Pers Med. 2021;**11**(11):1229

[89] Hogg JC, Chu F, Utokaparch S, Woods R, Elliott WM, Buzatu L, et al. The nature of small-airway obstruction in chronic obstructive pulmonary disease. The New England Journal of Medicine. 2004;**350**(26):2645-2653

[90] Barnes PJ. Corticosteroid resistance in patients with asthma and chronic obstructive pulmonary disease. The Journal of Allergy and Clinical Immunology. 2013;**131**(3):636-645

[91] Plichta J, Panek M. Role of the TGF-β cytokine and its gene polymorphisms in asthma etiopathogenesis. Frontiers in Allergy. 2025;**6**:1529071

[92] Nakamura R, Mukudai S, Bing R, Garabedian MJ, Branski RC. Complex fibroblast response to glucocorticoids may underlie variability of clinical efficacy in the vocal folds. Scientific Reports. 2020;**10**(1):20458

[93] Xiong DJP, Martin JG, Lauzon AM. Airway smooth muscle function in asthma. Frontiers in Physiology. 2022;**13**:993406

[94] Tran TN, Chen S, Emmanuel B, Altraja A, Bourdin A, Sheu CC, et al. Real-world biologic use patterns in severe asthma, 2015-2021: The CLEAR study. Pragmatic and Observational Research. 2025;**16**:51-66

[95] Nagase H, Suzukawa M, Oishi K, Matsunaga K. Biologics for severe asthma: The real-world evidence, effectiveness of switching, and prediction factors for the efficacy. Allergology International. 2023;**72**(1):11-23

[96] Singh S, Dutta J, Ray A, Karmakar A, Mabalirajan U. Airway epithelium: A neglected but crucial cell type in asthma pathobiology. Diagnostics (Basel). 2023;**13**(4):808

[97] O'Dwyer DN, Moore BB. The role of periostin in lung fibrosis and airway remodeling. Cellular and Molecular Life Sciences. 2017;**74**(23):4305-4314

[98] Tiotiu A. Biomarkers in asthma: State of the art. Asthma Research and Practice. 2018;**4**:10

[99] Faria N, Costa MI, Fernandes AL, Fernandes A, Fernandes B, Machado DC, et al. Biologic therapies for severe asthma: Current insights and future directions. Journal of Clinical Medicine [Internet]. 2025;**14**(9):3153

[100] Banno A, Reddy AT, Lakshmi SP, Reddy RC. Bidirectional interaction of airway epithelial remodeling and inflammation in asthma. Clinical Science (London, England). 2020;**134**(9):1063-1079

[101] Paik SS, Lee JM, Ko IG, Kim SR, Kang SW, An J, et al. Pirfenidone alleviates inflammation and fibrosis of acute respiratory distress syndrome by modulating the transforming growth factor-β/Smad signaling pathway. International Journal of Molecular Sciences. 2024;**25**(15):8014

[102] Lee J, Rhee CK, Lee JH, Yoon HJ, Kim IK, Hur J, et al. Effect of nintedanib on airway inflammation in a mouse model of acute asthma. The Journal of Asthma. 2020;**57**(1):11-20

[103] Lee HY, Hur J, Kim IK, Kang JY, Yoon HK, Lee SY, et al. Effect of nintedanib on airway inflammation and remodeling in a murine chronic asthma model. Experimental Lung Research. 2017;**43**(4-5):187-196

[104] Szefler S, Corren J, Silverberg JI, Okragly A, Sun Z, Natalie CR, et al. Lebrikizumab decreases type 2 inflammatory biomarker levels in patients with asthma: Data from randomized phase 3 trials (LAVOLTA I and II). Immunotherapy. 2024;**16**(20-22):1211-1216

[105] Baverel PG, White N, Vicini P, Karlsson MO, Agoram B. Dose-exposure-response relationship of the investigational anti-Interleukin-13 monoclonal antibody tralokinumab in patients with severe, uncontrolled asthma. Clinical Pharmacology and Therapeutics. 2018;**103**(5):826-835

[106] Menzies-Gow A, Corren J, Bourdin A, Chupp G, Israel E, Wechsler ME, et al. Tezepelumab in adults and adolescents with severe, uncontrolled asthma. The New England Journal of Medicine. 2021;**384**(19):1800-1809

[107] Kraik K, Tota M, Laska J, Łacwik J, Paździerz Ł, Sędek Ł, et al. The role of transforming growth factor-β (TGF-β) in Asthma and chronic obstructive pulmonary disease (COPD). Cells. 2024;**13**(15):1271

[108] Parker JM, Glaspole IN, Lancaster LH, Haddad TJ, She D, Roseti SL, et al. A phase 2 randomized controlled study of tralokinumab in subjects with idiopathic pulmonary fibrosis. American Journal of Respiratory and Critical Care Medicine. 2018;**197**(1):94-103

[109] Maher TM, Costabel U, Glassberg MK, Kondoh Y, Ogura T, Scholand MB, et al. Phase 2 trial to assess lebrikizumab in patients with idiopathic pulmonary fibrosis. The European Respiratory Journal. 2021;**57**(2):1902442

[110] Sridhar S, Zhao W, Pham T-H, Kearley J, White WI, Wu Y, et al. Tezepelumab decreases matrix remodelling and inflammatory pathways in patients with asthma. European Respiratory Journal. 2019;**54**(suppl 63):RCT3785

[111] Peng D, Fu M, Wang M, Wei Y, Wei X. Targeting TGF-β signal transduction for fibrosis and cancer therapy. Molecular Cancer. 2022;**21**(1):104

[112] Zhang T, Wang XF, Wang ZC, Lou D, Fang QQ, Hu YY, et al. Current potential therapeutic strategies targeting the TGF-beta/Smad signaling pathway to attenuate keloid and hypertrophic scar formation. Biomedicine & Pharmacotherapy. 2020;**129**:110287

[113] Sharma S, Yang IV, Schwartz DA. Epigenetic regulation of immune function in asthma. The Journal of Allergy and Clinical Immunology. 2022;**150**(2):259-265

[114] Chung FT, Huang HY, Lo CY, Huang YC, Lin CW, He CC, et al. Increased ratio of matrix metalloproteinase-9 (MMP-9)/tissue inhibitor metalloproteinase-1 from alveolar macrophages in chronic asthma with a fast decline in FEV(1) at 5-year follow-up. Journal of Clinical Medicine. 2019;**8**(9):1451

[115] Corbel M, Caulet-Maugendre S, Germain N, Molet S, Lagente V, Boichot E. Inhibition of bleomycin-induced pulmonary fibrosis in mice by the matrix metalloproteinase inhibitor batimastat. The Journal of Pathology. 2001;**193**(4):538-545

[116] Young TL, Mostovenko E, Denson JL, Begay JG, Lucas SN, Herbert G, et al. Pulmonary delivery of the broad-spectrum matrix metalloproteinase inhibitor marimastat diminishes multiwalled carbon nanotube-induced circulating bioactivity without reducing pulmonary inflammation. Particle and Fibre Toxicology. 2021;**18**(1):34

[117] Chalasani N, Abdelmalek MF, Garcia-Tsao G, Vuppalanchi R, Alkhouri N, Rinella M, et al. Effects of belapectin, an inhibitor of galectin-3, in patients with nonalcoholic steatohepatitis with cirrhosis and portal hypertension. Gastroenterology. 2020;**158**(5):1334-45 e5

[118] Hirani N, MacKinnon AC, Nicol L, Ford P, Schambye H, Pedersen A, et al. Target inhibition of galectin-3 by inhaled TD139 in patients with idiopathic pulmonary fibrosis. The European Respiratory Journal. 2021;**57**(5):2002559

[119] Ismail R, Habib HA, Anter AF, Amin A, Heeba GH. Modified citrus pectin ameliorates methotrexate-induced hepatic and pulmonary toxicity: Role of Nrf2, galectin-3/TLR-4/NF-kappaB/TNF-alpha and TGF-beta signaling pathways. Frontiers in Pharmacology. 2025;**16**:1528978

[120] Odun-Ayo F, Reddy L. Potential roles of modified pectin targeting galectin-3 against severe acute respiratory syndrome coronavirus-2. J. 2021;**4**(4):824-837

[121] Akkoc T, O'Mahony L, Ferstl R, Akdis C, Akkoc T. Mouse models of asthma: Characteristics, limitations and future perspectives on clinical translation. Advances in Experimental Medicine and Biology. 2022;**1376**:119-133

[122] Alessandrini F, Musiol S, Schneider E, Blanco-Perez F, Albrecht M. Mimicking antigen-driven asthma in rodent models-how close can we get? Frontiers in Immunology. 2020;**11**:575936

[123] Carroll OR, Pillar AL, Brown AC, Feng M, Chen H, Donovan C. Advances in respiratory physiology in mouse models of experimental asthma. Frontiers in Physiology. 2023;**14**:1099719

[124] Mullane K, Williams M. Animal models of asthma: Reprise or reboot? Biochemical Pharmacology. 2014;**87**(1):131-139

[125] Kumar RK, Herbert C, Foster PS. The "classical" ovalbumin challenge model of asthma in mice. Current Drug Targets. 2008;**9**(6):485-494

[126] Haspeslagh E, Debeuf N, Hammad H, Lambrecht BN. Murine models of allergic asthma. Methods in Molecular Biology. 2017;**1559**:121-136

[127] Blyth DI, Pedrick MS, Savage TJ, Hessel EM, Fattah D. Lung inflammation and epithelial changes in a murine model of atopic asthma. American Journal of Respiratory Cell and Molecular Biology. 1996;**14**(5):425-438

[128] Kumar RK, Herbert C, Foster PS. Expression of growth factors by airway epithelial cells in a model of chronic asthma: Regulation and relationship to subepithelial fibrosis. Clinical and Experimental Allergy. 2004;**34**(4):567-575

[129] An G, Wang W, Zhang X, Huang Q, Li Q, Chen S, et al. Combined blockade of IL-25, IL-33 and TSLP mediates amplified inhibition of airway inflammation and remodelling in a murine model of asthma. Respirology. 2020;**25**(6):603-612

[130] Zuhdi Alimam M, Piazza FM, Selby DM, Letwin N, Huang L, Rose MC. Muc-5/5ac mucin messenger RNA and protein expression is a marker of goblet cell metaplasia in murine airways. American Journal of Respiratory Cell and Molecular Biology. 2000;**22**(3):253-260

[131] Woo LN, Guo WY, Wang X, Young A, Salehi S, Hin A, et al. A 4-week model of house dust mite (HDM) induced allergic airways inflammation with airway remodeling. Scientific Reports. 2018;**8**(1):6925

[132] Allen IC. Induction of allergic airway disease using house dust mite allergen. Methods in Molecular Biology. 2013;**1032**:159-172

[133] Abu Khweek A, Kim E, Joldrichsen MR, Amer AO, Boyaka PN. Insights into mucosal innate immune responses in house dust mite-mediated allergic asthma. Frontiers in Immunology. 2020;**11**:534501

[134] Ruscitti F, Ravanetti F, Essers J, Ridwan Y, Belenkov S, Vos W, et al. Longitudinal assessment of bleomycin-induced lung fibrosis by micro-CT correlates with histological evaluation in mice. Multidisciplinary Respiratory Medicine. 2017;**12**:8

[135] Redente EF, Black BP, Backos DS, Bahadur AN, Humphries SM, Lynch DA, et al. Persistent, progressive pulmonary fibrosis and epithelial remodeling in mice. American Journal of Respiratory Cell and Molecular Biology. 2021;**64**(6):669-676

[136] Gul A, Yang F, Xie C, Du W, Mohammadtursun N, Wang B, et al. Pulmonary fibrosis model of mice induced by different administration methods of bleomycin. BMC Pulmonary Medicine. 2023;**23**(1):91

[137] Mouratis MA, Aidinis V. Modeling pulmonary fibrosis with bleomycin. Current Opinion in Pulmonary Medicine. 2011;**17**(5):355-361

[138] Redente EF, Jacobsen KM, Solomon JJ, Lara AR, Faubel S, Keith RC, et al. Age and sex dimorphisms contribute to the severity of bleomycin-induced lung injury and fibrosis. American Journal of Physiology. Lung Cellular and Molecular Physiology. 2011;**301**(4):L510-L518

[139] Lee CM, Park JW, Cho WK, Zhou Y, Han B, Yoon PO, et al. Modifiers of TGF-β1 effector function as novel therapeutic targets of pulmonary fibrosis. The Korean Journal of Internal Medicine. 2014;**29**(3):281-290

[140] Zhu Z, Homer RJ, Wang Z, Chen Q, Geba GP, Wang J, et al. Pulmonary

expression of interleukin-13 causes inflammation, mucus hypersecretion, subepithelial fibrosis, physiologic abnormalities, and eotaxin production. The Journal of Clinical Investigation. 1999;**103**(6):779-788

[141] Povedano JM, Martinez P, Flores JM, Mulero F, Blasco MA. Mice with pulmonary fibrosis driven by telomere dysfunction. Cell Reports. 2015;**12**(2):286-299

[142] Strobel B, Klein H, Leparc G, Stierstorfer BE, Gantner F, Kreuz S. Time and phenotype-dependent transcriptome analysis in AAV-TGFbeta1 and bleomycin-induced lung fibrosis models. Scientific Reports. 2022;**12**(1):12190

[143] Bormann T, Maus R, Stolper J, Tort Tarres M, Brandenberger C, Wedekind D, et al. Role of matrix metalloprotease-2 and MMP-9 in experimental lung fibrosis in mice. Respiratory Research. 2022;**23**(1):180

[144] Dong J, Ma Q. TIMP1 promotes multi-walled carbon nanotube-induced lung fibrosis by stimulating fibroblast activation and proliferation. Nanotoxicology. 2017;**11**(1):41-51

[145] Namvar S, Labram B, Rowley J, Herrick S. Aspergillus fumigatus-host interactions mediating airway wall remodelling in asthma. Journal of Fungi (Basel). 2022;**8**(2):159

[146] Al-Harbi NO, Nadeem A, Ahmad SF, AlThagfan SS, Alqinyah M, Alqahtani F, et al. Sulforaphane treatment reverses corticosteroid resistance in a mixed granulocytic mouse model of asthma by upregulation of antioxidants and attenuation of Th17 immune responses in the airways. European Journal of Pharmacology. 2019;**855**:276-284

[147] Daines M, Pereira R, Cunningham A, Pryor B, Besselsen DG, Liu Y, et al. Novel mouse models of fungal asthma. Frontiers in Cellular and Infection Microbiology. 2021;**11**:683194

[148] Ye W, Chen Q. Potential applications and perspectives of humanized mouse models. Annual Review of Animal Biosciences. 2022;**10**:395-417

[149] Doloff JC, Ma M, Sadraei A, Tam HH, Farah S, Hollister-Lock J, et al. Identification of a humanized mouse model for functional testing of immune-mediated biomaterial foreign body response. Science Advances. 2023;**9**(24):eade9488

[150] Acciani TH, Brandt EB, Khurana Hershey GK, Le Cras TD. Diesel exhaust particle exposure increases severity of allergic asthma in young mice. Clinical and Experimental Allergy. 2013;**43**(12):1406-1418

[151] Luthers CR, Dunn TM, Snow AL. ORMDL3 and asthma: Linking sphingolipid regulation to altered T cell function. Frontiers in Immunology. 2020;**11**:597945

[152] Ketelaar ME, Portelli MA, Dijk FN, Shrine N, Faiz A, Vermeulen CJ, et al. Phenotypic and functional translation of IL33 genetics in asthma. The Journal of Allergy and Clinical Immunology. 2021;**147**(1):144-157

[153] Janitri V, ArulJothi KN, Ravi Mythili VM, Singh SK, Prasher P, Gupta G, et al. The roles of patient-derived xenograft models and artificial intelligence toward precision medicine. MedComm 2020. 2024;**5**(10):e745

[154] Giarratana AO, Prendergast CM, Salvatore MM, Capaccione KM. TGF-beta signaling: Critical nexus of

fibrogenesis and cancer. Journal of Translational Medicine. 2024;**22**(1):594

[155] Wnuk D, Paw M, Ryczek K, Bochenek G, Sladek K, Madeja Z, et al. Enhanced asthma-related fibroblast to myofibroblast transition is the result of profibrotic TGF-beta/Smad2/3 pathway intensification and antifibrotic TGF-beta/Smad1/5/(8)9 pathway impairment. Scientific Reports. 2020;**10**(1):16492

[156] Le AV, Cho JY, Miller M, McElwain S, Golgotiu K, Broide DH. Inhibition of allergen-induced airway remodeling in Smad 3-deficient mice. Journal of Immunology. 2007;**178**(11):7310-7316

[157] Sebe A, Leivonen SK, Fintha A, Masszi A, Rosivall L, Kahari VM, et al. Transforming growth factor-beta-induced alpha-smooth muscle cell actin expression in renal proximal tubular cells is regulated by p38beta mitogen-activated protein kinase, extracellular signal-regulated protein kinase1,2 and the Smad signalling during epithelial-myofibroblast transdifferentiation. Nephrology, Dialysis, Transplantation. 2008;**23**(5):1537-1545

[158] Li C, Zhen G, Chai Y, Xie L, Crane JL, Farber E, et al. RhoA determines lineage fate of mesenchymal stem cells by modulating CTGF-VEGF complex in extracellular matrix. Nature Communications. 2016;**7**:11455

[159] Kaviratne M, Hesse M, Leusink M, Cheever AW, Davies SJ, McKerrow JH, et al. IL-13 activates a mechanism of tissue fibrosis that is completely TGF-beta independent. Journal of Immunology. 2004;**173**(6):4020-4029

[160] Jutzi JS, Mullally A. Two to tango! IL-13 and TGF-beta drive myelofibrosis. Blood. 2022;**140**(26):2767-2768

[161] Sidhu SS, Yuan S, Innes AL, Kerr S, Woodruff PG, Hou L, et al. Roles of epithelial cell-derived periostin in TGF-beta activation, collagen production, and collagen gel elasticity in asthma. Proceedings of the National Academy of Sciences of the United States of America. 2010;**107**(32):14170-14175

[162] Sun Z, Ji N, Ma Q, Zhu R, Chen Z, Wang Z, et al. Epithelial-mesenchymal transition in asthma airway remodeling is regulated by the IL-33/CD146 axis. Frontiers in Immunology. 2020;**11**:1598

[163] Claudio E, Wang H, Kamenyeva O, Tang W, Ha HL, Siebenlist U. IL-25 orchestrates activation of Th cells via conventional dendritic cells in tissue to exacerbate chronic house dust mite-induced asthma pathology. Journal of Immunology. 2019;**203**(8):2319-2327

[164] Habermann AC, Gutierrez AJ, Bui LT, Yahn SL, Winters NI, Calvi CL, et al. Single-cell RNA sequencing reveals profibrotic roles of distinct epithelial and mesenchymal lineages in pulmonary fibrosis. Science Advances. 2020;**6**(28):eaba1972

[165] Tan J, Tedrow JR, Nouraie M, Dutta JA, Miller DT, Li X, et al. Loss of twist1 in the mesenchymal compartment promotes increased fibrosis in experimental lung injury by enhanced expression of CXCL12. Journal of Immunology. 2017;**198**(6):2269-2285

[166] Gajjala PR, Kasam RK, Soundararajan D, Sinner D, Huang SK, Jegga AG, et al. Dysregulated overexpression of Sox9 induces fibroblast activation in pulmonary fibrosis. JCI Insight. 2021;**6**(20):e152503

[167] McMillan SJ, Lloyd CM. Prolonged allergen challenge in mice leads to persistent airway remodelling.

Clinical and Experimental Allergy. 2004;**34**(3):497-507

[168] Liu F, Lagares D, Choi KM, Stopfer L, Marinkovic A, Vrbanac V, et al. Mechanosignaling through YAP and TAZ drives fibroblast activation and fibrosis. American Journal of Physiology. Lung Cellular and Molecular Physiology. 2015;**308**(4):L344-L357

[169] Henderson J, O'Reilly S. The emerging role of metabolism in fibrosis. Trends in Endocrinology and Metabolism. 2021;**32**(8):639-653

[170] Tomlinson KL, Davies GC, Sutton DJ, Palframan RT. Neutralisation of interleukin-13 in mice prevents airway pathology caused by chronic exposure to house dust mite. PLoS One. 2010;**5**(10):e13136

[171] Lin SC, Chou HC, Chiang BL, Chen CM. CTGF upregulation correlates with MMP-9 level in airway remodeling in a murine model of asthma. Archives of Medical Science. 2017;**13**(3):670-676

[172] Li M, Krishnaveni MS, Li C, Zhou B, Xing Y, Banfalvi A, et al. Epithelium-specific deletion of TGF-β receptor type II protects mice from bleomycin-induced pulmonary fibrosis. The Journal of Clinical Investigation. 2011;**121**(1):277-287

[173] Rock JR, Barkauskas CE, Cronce MJ, Xue Y, Harris JR, Liang J, et al. Multiple stromal populations contribute to pulmonary fibrosis without evidence for epithelial to mesenchymal transition. Proceedings of the National Academy of Sciences of the United States of America. 2011;**108**(52):E1475-E1483

[174] Monticelli LA, Sonnenberg GF, Abt MC, Alenghat T, Ziegler CG, Doering TA, et al. Innate lymphoid cells promote lung-tissue homeostasis after infection with influenza virus. Nature Immunology. 2011;**12**(11):1045-1054

[175] Moore BB, Hogaboam CM. Murine models of pulmonary fibrosis. American Journal of Physiology. Lung Cellular and Molecular Physiology. 2008;**294**(2):L152-L160

[176] Pennati F, Leo L, Ferrini E, Sverzellati N, Bernardi D, Stellari FF, et al. Micro-CT-derived ventilation biomarkers for the longitudinal assessment of pathology and response to therapy in a mouse model of lung fibrosis. Scientific Reports. 2023;**13**(1):4462

[177] Castro JMA, Russo M. Use and limitations of noninvasive and invasive methods for studying pulmonary function. Drug Discovery Today: Disease Models. 2019;**29-30**:3-9

[178] Swonger JM, Liu JS, Ivey MJ, Tallquist MD. Genetic tools for identifying and manipulating fibroblasts in the mouse. Differentiation. 2016;**92**(3):66-83

[179] Yamaguchi T, Kato Y, Okuda T, Rokushima M, Izawa T, Kuwamura M, et al. Visualization of specific collagen-producing cells by Col1-GFP transgenic mice revealed novel type I collagen-producing cells other than fibroblasts in systemic organs/tissues. Biochemical and Biophysical Research Communications. 2018;**505**(1):267-273

[180] Magness ST, Bataller R, Yang L, Brenner DA. A dual reporter gene transgenic mouse demonstrates heterogeneity in hepatic fibrogenic cell populations. Hepatology. 2004;**40**(5):1151-1159

[181] Suzuki M, Ototake Y, Akita A, Asami M, Ikeda N, Watanabe T, et al. Periostin-An inducer of pro-fibrotic

phenotype in monocytes and monocyte-derived macrophages in systemic sclerosis. PLoS One. 2023;**18**(8):e0281881

[182] Wang F, Jin L, Wang X, Cui B, Yang Y, Duggan L, et al. Novel integration of spatial and single-cell omics data sets enables deeper insights into IPF pathogenesis. Proteomes. 2025;**13**(1):3

[183] Parkinson JE, Ghafoor M, Dodd RJ, Tompkins HE, Fergie M, Rattray M, et al. Extracellular matrix phenotyping by imaging mass cytometry defines distinct cellular matrix environments associated with allergic airway inflammation. bioRxiv 2024.11.15.623782. DOI: 10.1101/2024.11.15.623782

[184] Arif M, Basu A, Wolf KM, Park JK, Pommerolle L, Behee M, et al. An integrative multiomics framework for identification of therapeutic targets in pulmonary fibrosis. Advanced Science (Weinh). 2023;**10**(16):e2207454

[185] Rydell-Tormanen K, Johnson JR. The applicability of mouse models to the study of human disease. Methods in Molecular Biology. 2019;**1940**:3-22

[186] Lee JJ, Jacobsen EA, Ochkur SI, McGarry MP, Condjella RM, Doyle AD, et al. Human versus mouse eosinophils: "that which we call an eosinophil, by any other name would stain as red". The Journal of Allergy and Clinical Immunology. 2012;**130**(3):572-584

[187] Hammad H, Lambrecht BN. The basic immunology of asthma. Cell. 2021;**184**(6):1469-1485

[188] Kumar RK, Foster PS. Are mouse models of asthma appropriate for investigating the pathogenesis of airway hyper-responsiveness? Frontiers in Physiology. 2012;**3**:312

[189] Cho JY. Recent advances in mechanisms and treatments of airway remodeling in asthma: A message from the bench side to the clinic. The Korean Journal of Internal Medicine. 2011;**26**(4):367-383

[190] Vanoirbeek JA, Rinaldi M, De Vooght V, Haenen S, Bobic S, Gayan-Ramirez G, et al. Noninvasive and invasive pulmonary function in mouse models of obstructive and restrictive respiratory diseases. American Journal of Respiratory Cell and Molecular Biology. 2010;**42**(1):96-104

[191] Epstein MM, Tilp C, Erb KJ. The use of mouse asthma models to successfully discover and develop novel drugs. International Archives of Allergy and Immunology. 2017;**173**(2):61-70

[192] Darren JF, John VB, Alastair GS. Extracellular matrix, integrins, and mesenchymal cell function in the airways. Current Drug Targets. 2006;7(5):567-577

[193] Vladyslava VK. Matrix metalloproteinases as markers of respiratory tract remodeling and potential therapeutic target in patients with bronchial asthma. Eastern Ukrainian Medical Journal. 2021;**9**(2):174-188

[194] Stokes JR, Casale TB. Characterization of asthma endotypes: Implications for therapy. Annals of Allergy, Asthma & Immunology. 2016;**117**(2):121-125

[195] Gyorfi AH, Matei AE, Distler JHW. Targeting TGF-beta signaling for the treatment of fibrosis. Matrix Biology. 2018;**68-69**:8-27

[196] Scott G, Asrat S, Allinne J, Keat Lim W, Nagashima K, Birchard D, et al. IL-4 and IL-13, not eosinophils, drive

type 2 airway inflammation, remodeling and lung function decline. Cytokine. 2023;**162**:156091

[197] Sahnoon L, Bajbouj K, Mahboub B, Hamoudi R, Hamid Q. Targeting IL-13 and IL-4 in asthma: Therapeutic implications on airway remodeling in severe asthma. Clinical Reviews in Allergy and Immunology. 2025;**68**(1):44

[198] Izuhara K, Conway SJ, Moore BB, Matsumoto H, Holweg CT, Matthews JG, et al. Roles of periostin in respiratory disorders. American Journal of Respiratory and Critical Care Medicine. 2016;**193**(9):949-956

[199] Bonnesen B, Jensen J-US, Mathioudakis AG, Corlateanu A, Sivapalan P. Promising treatment biomarkers in asthma. Frontiers in Drug Safety and Regulation. 2023;**3**:1291471

[200] Amin K, Janson C, Bystrom J. Role of eosinophil granulocytes in allergic airway inflammation endotypes. Scandinavian Journal of Immunology. 2016;**84**(2):75-85

[201] Aceves SS, Broide DH. Airway fibrosis and angiogenesis due to eosinophil trafficking in chronic asthma. Current Molecular Medicine. 2008;**8**(5):350-358

[202] Sun Y, Shi Z, Liu B, Li X, Li G, Yang F, et al. YKL-40 mediates airway remodeling in asthma via activating FAK and MAPK signaling pathway. Cell Cycle. 2020;**19**(11):1378-1390

[203] Lai T, Wu D, Chen M, Cao C, Jing Z, Huang L, et al. YKL-40 expression in chronic obstructive pulmonary disease: Relation to acute exacerbations and airway remodeling. Respiratory Research. 2016;**17**:31

[204] Declercq J, Hammad H, Lambrecht BN, Smole U. Chitinases and chitinase-like proteins in asthma. Seminars in Immunology. 2023;**67**:101759

[205] Konradsen JR, James A, Nordlund B, Reinius LE, Soderhall C, Melen E, et al. The chitinase-like protein YKL-40: A possible biomarker of inflammation and airway remodeling in severe pediatric asthma. The Journal of Allergy and Clinical Immunology. 2013;**132**(2):328-35 e5

[206] Liu G, Cooley MA, Jarnicki AG, Borghuis T, Nair PM, Tjin G, et al. Fibulin-1c regulates transforming growth factor-beta activation in pulmonary tissue fibrosis. JCI Insight. 2019;**4**(16):e124529

[207] Lau JY, Oliver BG, Baraket M, Beckett EL, Hansbro NG, Moir LM, et al. Fibulin-1 is increased in asthma--a novel mediator of airway remodeling? PLoS One. 2010;**5**(10):e13360

[208] Aldakheel FM, Thomas PS, Bourke JE, Matheson MC, Dharmage SC, Lowe AJ. Relationships between adult asthma and oxidative stress markers and pH in exhaled breath condensate: A systematic review. Allergy. 2016;**71**(6):741-757

[209] Suzukawa M, Ohta K, Sugimoto M, Ohshima N, Kobayashi N, Tashimo H, et al. Identification of exhaled volatile organic compounds that characterize asthma phenotypes: A J-VOCSA study. Allergology International. 2024;**73**(4):524-531

[210] Dragonieri S, Marco MD, Ahroud M, Quaranta VN, Portacci A, Iorillo I, et al. Electronic nose based analysis of exhaled volatile organic compounds spectrum reveals asthmatic shifts and consistency in controls

post-exercise and spirometry. Journal of Breath Research. 2024;**18**(3):6005

[211] Panek M, Stawiski K, Kaszkowiak M, Kuna P. Cytokine TGFβ gene polymorphism in asthma: TGF-related SNP analysis enhances the prediction of disease diagnosis (a case-control study with multivariable data-mining model development). Frontiers in Immunology. 2022;**13**:746360

[212] Cui L, Jia J, Ma C-F, Li S-Y, Wang Y-P, Guo X-M, et al. IL-13 polymorphisms contribute to the risk of asthma: A meta-analysis. Clinical Biochemistry. 2012;**45**(4):285-288

[213] Zhang T, Huang P, Qiu C. Progresses in epigenetic studies of asthma from the perspective of high-throughput analysis technologies: A narrative review. Annals of Translational Medicine. 2022;**10**(8):493

[214] Potaczek DP, Bazan-Socha S, Wypasek E, Wygrecka M, Garn H. Recent developments in the role of histone acetylation in asthma. International Archives of Allergy and Immunology. 2024;**185**(7):641-651

[215] Ricciardolo FLM, Carriero V, Bertolini F. Biomarkers in Asthma. In: Janes SM, editor. Encyclopedia of Respiratory Medicine. Second ed. Oxford: Academic Press; 2022. pp. 342-351

[216] Ntontsi P, Papathanassiou E, Loukides S, Bakakos P, Hillas G. Targeted anti-IL-13 therapies in asthma: Current data and future perspectives. Expert Opinion on Investigational Drugs. 2018;**27**(2):179-186

[217] Kim MA, Shin YS, Pham le D, Park HS. Adult asthma biomarkers. Current Opinion in Allergy and Clinical Immunology. 2014;**14**(1):49-54

[218] Rathnayake SNH, Van den Berge M, Faiz A. Genetic profiling for disease stratification in chronic obstructive pulmonary disease and asthma. Current Opinion in Pulmonary Medicine. 2019;**25**(3):317-322

[219] Xu S, Panettieri RA Jr, Jude J. Metabolomics in asthma: A platform for discovery. Molecular Aspects of Medicine. 2022;**85**:100990

[220] Pavord ID, Afzalnia S, Menzies-Gow A, Heaney LG. The current and future role of biomarkers in type 2 cytokine-mediated asthma management. Clinical and Experimental Allergy. 2017;**47**(2):148-160

[221] Parulekar AD, Atik MA, Hanania NA. Periostin, a novel biomarker of TH2-driven asthma. Current Opinion in Pulmonary Medicine. 2014;**20**(1):60-65

Section 3

Asthma in Allergy Clinics

Chapter 3

Evaluation of the Asthmatic Patient for Primary and Secondary Immunodeficiencies and Importance of Vaccinations in Asthma

Katarzyna Napiórkowska-Baran

Abstract

Asthma is a chronic inflammatory disease of the airways, the course of which can be significantly modified by the presence of primary (PIDs) and secondary immunodeficiencies (SIDs). The coexistence of these disorders affects the frequency of infections, severity of symptoms, and response to treatment. The purpose of this chapter is to comprehensively analyze the diagnosis of patients with asthma in terms of immune deficits, as well as to discuss the importance of prevention of infections, especially through immunization. The most important types of PIDs and SIDs, their clinical manifestations, and diagnostic methods are presented. The impact of immunosuppressive therapies, such as corticosteroids, on immune function and the risk of infection is also discussed. Special attention was paid to vaccination – its effectiveness, safety, and individualization depending on the type of immunodeficiency. The chapter emphasizes the need for a multidisciplinary approach in the care of patients with asthma and immune deficiencies and the importance of educating the patient and his immediate environment in the prevention of infection.

Keywords: asthma, primary immunodeficiencies, secondary immunodeficiencies, inborn errors of immunity, immunological diagnostics, vaccination, immunosuppression, respiratory tract infections

1. Introduction

Asthma is one of the most common chronic diseases that significantly affects patients' quality of life and their ability to function on a daily basis. Despite significant advances in the diagnosis and treatment of this disease, many aspects related to its pathogenesis and therapy, especially in patients with additional health burdens, remain a challenge for modern medicine. Of particular concern may be the issues of the coexistence of asthma with immunodeficiencies – both primary and secondary, which significantly modify the course of the disease, response to treatment, and patient's susceptibility to infection.

In the context of the increasing number of immunodeficiency diagnoses and the growing use of immunosuppressive therapies that secondarily affect immune system function, the importance of effective preventive strategies is growing. Vaccination plays a key role in this group of patients in preventing infections, which are important exacerbators of asthma. However, combining the diagnosis and treatment of asthma with an approach that targets immune deficiencies and infection prevention requires individualization, as well as consideration of the specific challenges unique to each patient group. In particular, analyzing the role of vaccination, its effectiveness, and safety in patients with different types of immunodeficiencies is an important part of optimizing medical care. The purpose of this chapter is to analyze the issues of diagnosis and treatment of patients with asthma in the context of primary and secondary immunodeficiencies and to assess the impact of vaccination on the course of the disease and the effectiveness of therapy.

2. Primary immunodeficiencies in patients with asthma

Primary immunodeficiencies (PIDs), now also called inborn errors of immunity (IEIs), are an important topic in the context of asthma, affecting patients' susceptibility to infections and disease complications. Analyzing the definition, classification, and most common clinical manifestations of these deficiencies allows us to understand how various immune defects can affect the course of asthma and its treatment. In addition, the diagnosis and identification of primary immunodeficiencies are becoming crucial for the effective management of patients' conditions. In the following chapter, the synonyms PIDs and IEIs will be used interchangeably.

2.1 Definition and classification of primary immunodeficiencies

Primary immunodeficiencies are a complex group of nearly 600 conditions whose pathogenesis is associated with genetic defects affecting various components of the immune system [1]. T lymphocytes, B lymphocytes, Natural killer (NK) cells, or the complement system can be affected, leading to diverse clinical manifestations, including recurrent infections and immune dysregulation [2]. A key aspect of PIDs is their impact on the immune system's ability to respond to infectious agents, resulting in susceptibility to bacterial, viral, fungal, or parasitic infections. In addition, these mechanisms can promote the development of chronic inflammation as well as autoimmune diseases, cancers, and allergies, highlighting the multidimensionality of the problem. Diagnosis of these conditions remains a significant challenge, requiring both detailed clinical analysis and advanced laboratory testing to identify molecular defects and their clinical consequences.

The classification of PIDs, developed by the International Union of Immunological Societies (IUIS), includes ten main categories, each reflecting distinct pathophysiological mechanisms (**Table 1**). Analysis and classification of PIDs is crucial to understanding the complexity of these conditions and adapting appropriate therapeutic strategies [1]. The 10 most common primary immunodeficiencies are listed in **Table 2**.

Immunodeficiencies affecting cellular and humoral immunity involve severe conditions in which both T lymphocytes (cellular immunity) and B lymphocytes (humoral immunity) are impaired. They often manifest in early childhood with

1. Immunodeficiencies affecting cellular and humoral immunity
2. Combined immunodeficiencies with associated or syndromic features
3. Predominantly antibody deficiencies
4. Diseases of immune dysregulation
5. Congenital defects of phagocyte number or function
6. Defects in intrinsic and innate immunity
7. Autoinflammatory disorders
8. Complement deficiencies
9. Bone marrow failure
10. Phenocopies of inborn errors of immunity

Table 1.
IEIs classification according to IUIS [1].

Warning Signs in Children
1. ≥ 4 new ear infections within 1 year. 2. ≥ 2 serious sinus infections within 1 year. 3. ≥ 2 months on antibiotics with little effect. 4. ≥ 2 cases of pneumonia within 1 year. 5. Failure of an infant to gain weight or grow normally. 6. Recurrent, deep skin, or organ abscesses. 7. Persistent thrush in mouth or fungal infection on skin. 8. Need for IV antibiotics to clear infections. 9. ≥ 2 deep-seated infections including septicemia. 10. 1A family history of PID.
Warning Signs in Adults
1. ≥ 2 new ear infections within 1 year. 2. ≥ 2 new sinus infections within 1 year, in the absence of allergy. 3. 1 case of pneumonia per year for >1 year. 4. Chronic diarrhea with weight loss. 5. Recurrent viral infections (colds, herpes, warts, condyloma). 6. Recurrent need for IV antibiotics to clear infections. 7. Recurrent, deep abscesses of the skin or internal organs. 8. Persistent thrush or fungal infection on skin or elsewhere. 9. Infection with normally harmless tuberculosis-like bacteria. 10. A family history of PID.

Table 2.
The Jeffrey Modell foundation's 10 warning signs of primary immune deficiency [3].

severe, recurrent infections and are particularly difficult to manage due to their high mortality without early intervention such as hematopoietic stem cell transplantation (HSCT). A classic example is severe combined immunodeficiency (SCID).

Combined immunodeficiencies with associated or syndromic features are immune deficiencies accompanied by manifestations in other organ systems (e.g., skin, nervous system, and skeletal system). Patients may present with developmental delays, dysmorphic features, or hearing loss. Examples include DiGeorge syndrome and Nijmegen breakage syndrome [4].

Predominantly antibody deficiencies are the most common group of IEIs, accounting for over 50% of all PIDs. They most frequently present with recurrent respiratory tract infections. Selective IgA deficiency, affecting approximately 1 in 500 individuals of Caucasian descent, is one of the most prevalent PIDs. Although often asymptomatic or mild, it is associated with an increased risk of mucosal infections, autoimmune diseases, and allergies. Another clinically significant deficiency in this group is common variable immunodeficiency (CVID), characterized by decreased levels of one or more immunoglobulin classes (IgG, IgA, and optionally IgM), along with impaired responses to vaccinations and infections. CVID exhibits considerable clinical variability and requires an individualized diagnostic and therapeutic approach, along with multidisciplinary care. Patients with CVID require lifelong IgG replacement therapy, either intravenously (IVIG) or subcutaneously (SCIG). In IgG subclass deficiency, the total IgG concentration may be normal, but there is a deficiency in one or more subclasses: IgG1, IgG2, IgG3, or IgG4. IgG2 and/or IgG4 deficiency is most commonly observed. This condition can occur in isolation or co-occur with other immune deficiencies, such as selective IgA deficiency. An interesting immunodeficiency is specific antibody deficiency (SAD). This is a type of primary immunodeficiency in which the patient has normal total immunoglobulin concentrations (IgG, IgA, and IgM) but fails to produce an adequate amount of antibodies in response to polysaccharide antigens, such as those found in pneumococcal vaccines. The concentrations of major immunoglobulin classes and subclasses are typically within the normal range, which may lead to diagnostic errors [5].

Diseases of immune dysregulation are characterized by abnormal control of immune responses, leading to autoimmunity, lymphoproliferation, or homeostatic imbalances. Examples include IPEX syndrome (immune dysregulation, polyendocrinopathy, enteropathy, and X-linked) and APECED (autoimmune polyendocrinopathy with candidiasis and ectodermal dystrophy).

Congenital defects of phagocyte number or function involve dysfunction of neutrophils or macrophages, resulting in impaired clearance of bacteria and fungi. Examples include chronic granulomatous disease (CGD) and severe congenital neutropenia.

Defects in intrinsic and innate immunity include abnormalities in pathogen recognition, such as impaired Toll-like receptor (TLR) signaling and disrupted antiviral responses. These defects typically result in severe viral or bacterial infections despite preserved adaptive immunity. An example is type I interferon deficiency.

Autoinflammatory disorders are characterized by recurrent inflammatory episodes in the absence of autoantibodies or autoreactive lymphocytes. Typical symptoms include fever, skin rashes, and joint pain. An example is familial Mediterranean fever (FMF).

Complement deficiencies involve impaired activation of the complement system, which increases susceptibility to infections (especially meningococcal) and autoimmune diseases. Examples include deficiencies of complement components C2, C3, and C5.

Bone marrow failure refers to a group of disorders in which the bone marrow fails to produce blood cells adequately, leading to pancytopenia. An example is Fanconi anemia.

Phenocopies of inborn errors of immunity are acquired clinical conditions that mimic IEIs but are not caused by inherited genetic defects. They may result from autoantibodies against cytokines (e.g., anti-IFN-γ antibodies), which are typical in adults with recurrent atypical infections [6, 7].

An analysis conducted by El-Sayed et al. and published in 2022 in the World Allergy Organization Journal demonstrated that allergic symptoms were the first manifestation of PID in 8% of patients and contributed to delayed diagnosis in approximately 7.5% of cases. The study included data from 30 centers across 23 countries, collectively caring for 8450 patients with PID, as well as from the United States Immunodeficiency Network (USIDNET), which covered 2332 patients. According to data from the international centers, allergies were reported in 16.3% of PID patients, with asthma (3.6%), atopic dermatitis (3.6%), and allergic rhinitis (3.0%) being the most common. According to USIDNET data, the overall prevalence of allergies among patients with IEI was 68.8%, with bronchial asthma observed in 46.9%. Allergies were most frequently associated with predominantly antibody deficiencies (40.3%; range 19.2–62.5%), followed by combined immunodeficiencies (20.0%; range 10–32%) [8].

In the study by Lee SH et al., the authors aimed to estimate the prevalence of PIDs and their impact on asthma exacerbations in adult patients. The retrospective study included 2866 adult asthma patients, of whom 157 (5.49%) met the diagnostic criteria for PID, primarily IgG3 subclass deficiency. These patients experienced significantly more frequent asthma exacerbations and had more severe disease (32.5 vs. 13% in the non-PID group). The risk of exacerbation was 1.7 times higher in the PID group. Intravenous immunoglobulin (IVIG) therapy was administered to 31.8% of patients with PID and proved effective in reducing the frequency of infections and exacerbations. The authors suggest that PID, particularly IgG3 deficiency, should be considered an important risk factor for asthma exacerbations in adults. Early detection and treatment of PID, including IVIG therapy, may improve asthma control and quality of life in these patients [9].

2.2 Diagnosis and most common clinical manifestations

The key to diagnosing PID is, first and foremost, considering the possibility of its occurrence. Early detection and treatment not only prevent the development of incurable organ changes in the future but, above all, prevent the patient's death.

The Jeffrey Modell Foundation (JMF) has created a list of 10 symptoms for both children and adults that may indicate the presence of congenital immunodeficiency. They are presented in **Table 2**. It should be remembered that the frequency of infections in children may be higher due to the immaturity of the immune system and attendance at a nursery or kindergarten. **Table 3** presents the clinical manifestations and typical pathogens depending on the type of deficiency.

Differential diagnosis of PID becomes particularly important in children with asthma who experience severe, recurrent lower respiratory tract infections. In such cases, the possibility that these infections are associated with immune deficiencies should be considered, especially in the context of poor response to standard asthma treatment. Prolonged lower respiratory tract infections in children may be the first sign of an immunological deficit, particularly in at-risk groups such as children with a family history of immunodeficiencies. Moreover, the high risk of rhinovirus infections and virus-associated wheezing in young children may justify a thorough diagnostic workup, especially in cases with atopic predisposition. Differential diagnosis must include comprehensive immunological testing as well as imaging studies. **Table 4** presents the diagnostic algorithm in case of suspected PID.

Type of ID	Key Cells/Systems	Typical Pathogens	Symptoms
Humoral (antibody-related)	B lymphocytes, antibodies (IgG, IgA, IgM)	*H. influenzae*, *S. pneumoniae*, *Enterovirus* sp.	Recurrent infections of ears, sinuses, bronchi, and lungs; gastrointestinal infections
Cellular	T lymphocytes	Viruses: *CMV, HSV, VZV* Fungi: *Candida* sp., *P. jirovecii;* Opportunistic Bacteria: *Mycobacterium* sp., *Listeria* sp.	Disseminated viral infections, severe fungal infections, opportunistic infections, diarrhea, growth failure
Phagocytic defects	Neutrophils, macrophages	*S. aureus*, *S. marcescens*, *Aspergillus* sp.	Skin and soft tissue abscesses, liver and lung infections
Complement Deficiency	Terminal pathway (C5–C9)	*N. meningitidis*	Recurrent meningitis and sepsis
	Classical pathway (C1q, C2, C4)	*S. pneumoniae, H. influenzae*	Respiratory infections
	C3 – central element of all activation pathways	*S. pneumoniae, H. influenzae*	Severe purulent infections

Abbreviations: CMV – Cytomegalovirus, H. influenzae – Haemophilus influenzae, HSV – Herpes Simplex Virus, ID – Immunodeficiencies, IgA – Immunoglobulin A, IgG – Immunoglobulin G, IgM – Immunoglobulin M, L. monocytogenes – Listeria monocytogenes, N. meningitidis – Neisseria meningitidis, P. jirovecii – Pneumocystis jirovecii, S. aureus – Staphylococcus aureus, S. marcescens – Serratia marcescens, S. pneumoniae – Streptococcus pneumoniae, VZV – Varicella Zoster Virus [6, 10].

Table 3.
Types of immunodeficiencies, key cells, pathogens, and symptoms.

Suspect primary immunodeficiencies based on the following findings in medical history:

- recurrent/prolonged and/or chronic/opportunistic infections,
- autoimmunity,
- hematologic disorders,
- malignancies,
- allergies (atypical and/or difficult to treat).

Exclude Secondary Immunodeficiencies

Perform the following tests:

- Complete blood count with manual differential and evaluate WBC and lymphocyte count – antibodies (i.e., immunoglobulins) are produced exclusively by B lymphocytes.
- Protein electrophoresis – total protein and γ-globulin fraction assessment:
  - o allows the detection of protein loss or secondary antibody deficiency
  - o immunoglobulins are mainly present in the γ-globulin fraction (all immunoglobulin classes) and to a lesser extent in the β-globulin fraction (IgA and IgM)
  - o in the case of deficiencies of single immunoglobulin classes, IgG subclass deficiency, or specific antibody deficiency, the result may be normal
- Serum levels of major immunoglobulin classes: IgA, IgG, IgM
  - o available in every commercial laboratory and most hospitals
  - o relatively low cost compared to other specialized tests
  - o secondary immunodeficiencies should be excluded (see **Table 5**)
  - o remember that reference ranges vary by age

Refer the patient to the Immunology Outpatient Clinic or Immunology Clinic
If possible, perform the recommended tests: • Assessment of humoral immunity: o IgG subclass levels o Isohemagglutinin titers (anti-A, anti-B) – can be performed in every blood donation center o Specific antibody titers to previously administered vaccines (tetanus, diphtheria) o Specific antibody titers after pneumococcal vaccination (in children >2 years) o Lymphocyte phenotyping – helps determine the number of B lymphocytes • Assessment of cellular immunity: o Delayed-type hypersensitivity test – tuberculin skin test (TST) o Lymphocyte transformation test (LTT, mitogen-induced proliferation) o Natural killer (NK) cell cytotoxicity assay • Assessment of phagocytic cells: o Production of reactive oxygen species (ROS) – NBT test (Nitroblue Tetrazolium) o Expression of adhesion molecules – flow cytometry o Assessment of chemotaxis o Assessment of particle uptake and phagocytosis • Assessment of the complement system: o Total hemolytic complement activity: CH50 o Alternative hemolytic complement activity: AH50 o C1 esterase inhibitor deficiency o Concentration of specific complement components o Genetic tests

Table 4.
Diagnostic algorithm in case of suspected PID [11].

Last and first name:		
MEDICAL HISTORY		
Parameter	**Yes**	**No**
Age		
• < 16 years of age	☐	☐
• > 65 years of age	☐	☐
Chronic diseases		
• Type 2 diabetes mellitus	☐	☐
• Chronic kidney disease	☐	☐
• Rheumatological disease	☐	☐
• Inflammatory bowel disease	☐	☐
• Other autoimmune disease	☐	☐
• Neoplasms	☐	☐
• Liver diseases	☐	☐
• Pancreas diseases	☐	☐
• Chronic infections	☐	☐
• Other	☐	☐

Last and first name:		
Medicaments		
• Immunosuppressive medications	☐	☐
• Other	☐	☐
Nutritional status		
• Malnutrition	☐	☐
• Normal weight	☐	☐
• Overweight	☐	☐
• Obesity	☐	☐
Deficiency of non-nutritive bioactive compounds (e.g. extensive information about the diet used)		
• Suspected deficiency	☐	☐
Addiction		
• Alcohol	☐	☐
• Drugs	☐	☐
• Medicines	☐	☐
• Other	☐	☐
Stress coping assessment		
• Very good	☐	☐
• Satisfactory	☐	☐
• Unsatisfactory	☐	☐
Other information		
• For example, hereditary diseases (including primary immunodeficiencies)	☐	☐
ADDITIONAL TESTS		
• morphology with smear		
• concentrations of the main immunoglobulin classes (IgA, IgG, and IgM)		
• allergy tests		
• assesses nutrient deficiencies: vitamin D, folic acid, vitamin B12, iron, total iron binding capacity (TIBC), ferritin, and albumin		
• bronchoscopy		
• microbiological tests, for example, sputum culture		
• imaging tests – X-ray, CT (in the case of uncontrolled asthma, difficult-to-treat asthma, and suspected complications, e.g., bronchiectasis)		

Table 5.
Secondary immunodeficiencies diagnostic scheme [12].

3. Secondary immunodeficiencies in patients with asthma

The impact of secondary immunodeficiencies (SIDs) on patients with asthma is becoming increasingly apparent in an epidemiological and clinical context. This chapter highlights how secondary immunodeficiencies can affect patients' susceptibility to infection, disease exacerbations, and the effectiveness of therapies, emphasizing the importance of a holistic approach to patient care.

3.1 Causes and diagnosis of secondary immunodeficiencies

Secondary immunodeficiencies in asthma patients may have multiple causes, which include chronic diseases, malnutrition, infections, cancer, and medical interventions such as immunosuppressive therapies. The causes of SIDs are shown in **Table 6**.

The proper functioning of the immune system depends not only on genetic factors and comorbidities but also on whether the building blocks for the synthesis of its components are provided. A proper diet should provide all the necessary nutrients such as carbohydrates, proteins, and fats but also non-nutritional bioactive compounds. The latter include, among others, macroelements, microelements, and vitamins. Unfortunately, changes introduced in the food industry have caused a significant loss of components necessary for the proper functioning of the immune system. This is due, among other things, to the use of artificial fertilizers containing much less valuable ingredients than natural fertilizers and the consumption of highly processed food. For example, thiamine is found mainly in the bran and germ of wheat grains, and up to 50% of it is lost during milling. Fresh leafy vegetables stored at room temperature lose up to 70% of folic acid within 3 days [15, 16]. In the UK and other countries, a decrease in the content of essential minerals in fruits and vegetables has been noted. A new analysis of long-term trends in the mineral content of fruits and vegetables from three editions of the British Food Composition Tables (1940, 1991, and 2019) was carried out. Concentrations of all elements except phosphorus decreased between 1940 and 2019, with the largest overall reductions over this 80-year period being for Na (52%), Fe (50%), Cu (49%) and Mg (10%) [17]. Studies conducted by Geigy Pharmaceutical Company comparing vitamin

Category	Examples/Notes
Malnutrition and nutrient deficiencies	Deficiencies in vitamins and minerals (e.g., zinc and vitamin D)
Malignancies	Hematological and solid tumors
Infections	HIV, EBV, CMV, tuberculosis, bacterial infections
Hereditary and metabolic diseases	Down Syndrome, diabetes
Injuries and surgeries	Burns, extensive surgical procedures, splenectomy
Digestive tract diseases	Celiac disease and other enteropathies, Whipple's disease, inflammatory bowel disease, chronic inflammation and liver cirrhosis, chronic pancreatitis
Other Severe Diseases	Autoimmune diseases, uremia, and nephropathy, chronic kidney disease
Immunosuppressive drugs	Corticosteroids, chemotherapy, biological agents
Age-related	Premature infants, neonates, elderly
Pregnancy	Physiological immune modulation during gestation
Substance abuse	Alcohol, psychoactive drugs
Radiation exposure	UV radiation, ionizing radiation

Abbreviations: HIV – human immunodeficiency virus, EBV – Epstein-Barr Virus, CMV – cytomegalovirus [13, 14].

Table 6.
Causes of secondary immunodeficiencies [13, 14].

and mineral concentrations in selected plant foods between 1985 and 2002 showed significant decreases in calcium, magnesium, folate, vitamin B6, and vitamin C [18]. Unfortunately, the need for additional supplementation is underestimated by doctors who are unaware of the changes that have occurred in food over recent decades. On the part of patients, supplementation, if carried out, is often self-administered in an uncontrolled manner.

A simplified SID diagnostic scheme is presented in **Table 5**.

3.2 Impact on the course and treatment of asthma

In the context of asthma, patients with SID are more susceptible to lower respiratory tract infections and disease exacerbations, which are associated with a reduction or loss of immune function. Infections arising from these immune disturbances significantly enhance inflammatory responses in the airways, often leading to difficult-to-control asthma exacerbations [19]. Chronic conditions such as diabetes or respiratory infections increase the risk of secondary immune disturbances, highlighting the need to consider these factors in diagnosis and treatment. Special attention is given to immunosuppressive therapies, such as the use of corticosteroids, which affect the production of inflammatory cytokines, including type I interferons, thereby weakening antiviral defense and contributing to more frequent asthma exacerbations [20]. Rhinoviruses can trigger particularly intense inflammatory responses, resulting in more severe disease symptoms [19]. Minimizing corticosteroid doses, in accordance with the principle of using the lowest effective dose, combined with monitoring signs of infection, may improve asthma control and reduce the risk of infections in this group of patients. Chronic respiratory tract infections can lead to permanent structural changes in the lungs, resulting in long-term respiratory limitations [21]. Regular evaluations, such as spirometry, imaging tests and immunoglobulin level assessments, are essential for the functional assessment of the respiratory system in these patients, allowing for the early implementation of appropriate therapeutic interventions.

Immunosuppressive drugs, such as rituximab, have a specific impact on the immune system. Rituximab, an anti-CD20 monoclonal antibody, causes B cell depletion, resulting in decreased immunoglobulin levels and increased susceptibility to infections—particularly bacterial—that can significantly disrupt the course of asthma. In the case of mycophenolate mofetil, another immunosuppressive agent, its mechanism of action involves inhibition of T and B lymphocyte proliferation and reduction of cytotoxic T cell activity, which increases the risk of both viral and bacterial infections [14, 22]. For patients undergoing immunosuppressive therapy, close monitoring of their immune status is essential in order to minimize the risk of asthma exacerbations and severe infections.

Secondary immunodeficiencies significantly affect the efficacy of vaccines in patients with asthma, further increasing their susceptibility to infections and disease exacerbations. Polysaccharide vaccines, such as those against pneumococci, are among the most important strategies for preventing lower respiratory tract infections. However, their effectiveness may be limited in this patient group due to impaired immune responses. Patients with SID often require additional vaccine doses to enhance post-vaccination protection [22]. Monitoring antibody levels after vaccination allows for the adjustment of immunization schedules to meet individual patient needs, which in turn may reduce the risk of infection and improve asthma control.

Socioeconomic determinants of health, such as limited access to vaccination or biologic therapies, place an additional burden on individuals with SID from lower-income backgrounds. Among these populations, asthma exacerbations and infectious complications occur more frequently due to difficulties in accessing appropriate healthcare services [23]. Studies show that individuals from racial or ethnic minority groups are more likely to suffer from severe asthma and have restricted access to treatment, which significantly worsens their health outcomes [24]. The implementation of health policies ensuring equal access to modern therapies and vaccinations could substantially improve the prognosis of patients with SID and asthma [23].

In summary, secondary immunodeficiencies complicate asthma management and worsen disease control; however, the implementation of coordinated therapeutic and preventive strategies may help mitigate their negative impact.

4. Importance of vaccinations in patients with asthma and immunodeficiencies

Vaccinations play a key role in protecting patients with asthma from infections that can lead to exacerbations and complications. Understanding the importance of immunization in the context of their specific health needs is essential to improving quality of life and reducing the risk of infection. Collaboration with the healthcare team and monitoring the effectiveness of vaccinations are important components of the overall treatment strategy for patients with asthma and immunodeficiencies.

4.1 Recommended vaccinations

Vaccinations are a key element of infection prevention in patients with asthma, especially those with concomitant immunodeficiencies, but their use requires precise adjustment to the patient's immunological status. Inactivated vaccines are considered safe also in immunocompromised patients. In particular, vaccines against influenza and pneumococci show significant potential in reducing asthma exacerbations and the frequency of hospitalizations resulting from respiratory infections [25].

Their mechanism of action is based on the stimulation of the immune system to produce specific antibodies, which is particularly important in people with immune deficiencies exposed to lower respiratory tract infections. However, we cannot forget that vaccinations also stimulate the response of other types of immunity, including the very important cellular immunity, as well as the complement system. Although the effectiveness of inactivated vaccinations may be weakened in this group of patients, the benefits of vaccinations significantly outweigh the risk of potentially weaker immunomodulatory effects. It should also be remembered that in patients with asthma taking immunosuppressive drugs or patients with other immune deficiencies, monitoring antibody concentrations after immunization to confirm the adequacy of the immune response does not reflect the full potential of vaccinations.

Vaccination against influenza is particularly important from the point of view of prevention, as the influenza virus is one of the most common factors exacerbating the course of asthma, leading not only to severe respiratory complications but also to frequent hospitalizations of people with reduced immunity. In the case of patients with asthma and immunodeficiencies, the response to vaccination against influenza may be less intense than in healthy people, but the effectiveness of this solution in preventing influenza infections and their consequences remains an important element of the therapeutic strategy.

In turn, vaccination against pneumococci, which is one of the key methods of preventing bacterial infections of the lower respiratory tract, helps reduce the risk of pneumonia and sepsis, which are particularly dangerous in people with immunodeficiencies [25]. PCV13 (conjugated vaccine) and PPSV23 (polysaccharide vaccine) vaccines are recommended, especially for people with severe asthma or concomitant chronic diseases. These are supplementary vaccinations, and to obtain the most beneficial effect of vaccination, it is recommended to first perform PCV13 (single dose), and then after at least 8 weeks, PPSV23 vaccination, which should be repeated every 3–5 years. In the case of using the relatively recently introduced PCV20 vaccine, administration of the PPSV23 vaccine is no longer necessary [26].

In patients with asthma, it is also necessary to remember booster vaccinations against tetanus, diphtheria, and pertussis (Tdap), which should be performed in adults once every 10 years. In children, these are vaccinations included in the mandatory vaccination schedule.

Vaccination against respiratory syncytial virus (RSV) is considered in individual cases, especially in adults at high risk of severe infection. Asthma patients, due to their increased susceptibility to viral and bacterial infections, should also be included in vaccination programs against varicella zoster virus (VZV). The increased risk of VZV infection, which in the group of people with asthma is up to 24% compared to the general population, justifies the introduction of vaccination as a standard element of preventive care [27]. The recombinant version of the VZV vaccine, containing the viral glycoprotein gE and the AS01B adjuvant, shows a high efficacy of about 90%, even in the oldest age groups and in people with immunodeficiencies, making it the preferred choice for this group of patients [28].

Special recommendations apply to COVID-19 vaccinations in immunocompromised patients, especially those receiving immunosuppressive therapy. Lee's study showed that seroconversion after a single dose of mRNA vaccine may be insufficient, indicating the need for additional doses to improve the immune response. The second and third doses of the mRNA vaccine significantly increase seroconversion rates, which allows for better protection of patients against infection [29].

Live vaccines such as MMR (measles, mumps, and rubella), OPV (oral poliomyelitis vaccine), or BCG (tuberculosis vaccine) are contraindicated in patients with severe immunodeficiencies due to the risk of infection with attenuated pathogens [30]. In such cases, it is recommended to use inactivated vaccines, if possible, or to weigh the benefits and risks individually for the degree of immunodeficiency. In patients with milder immunological defects, decisions regarding live vaccinations should be made in consultation with the immunologist and the treating physician.

4.2 Contraindications to vaccination

An absolute, so-called permanent contraindication to all types of vaccines is a systemic anaphylactic reaction (e.g., anaphylactic shock, laryngeal edema, or anaphylaxis involving ≥2 organ systems) following a previous dose of the vaccine. However, it is important to distinguish an anaphylactic reaction from a fainting episode or panic attack after vaccination, which are not contraindications to further doses and occur much more frequently. Another contraindication is a systemic anaphylactic reaction to vaccine components, such as egg protein, neomycin, polyethylene glycol (PEG), or polysorbate 80.

Contraindications to the administration of live vaccines include congenital or acquired immune disorders (especially cellular), also resulting from radiotherapy, chemotherapy and immunosuppressive treatment, including GCS at a dose equivalent to >20 mg/day of prednisone for ≥14 days in individuals weighing >10 kg. Vaccination can be performed >1 month after the end of such GCS therapy. The use of local GCS preparations (on the skin, intranasally or inhaled) or physiological replacement doses (e.g., in adrenal insufficiency) is not a contraindication to vaccination. Live vaccines should not be administered to pregnant women 1–3 months before a planned pregnancy. The minimum interval between the administration of subsequent doses or different live vaccines is 4 weeks (this rule does not apply to the "live" oral vaccine against typhoid fever). During the same visit, several live vaccines can be administered – except in patients with immunodeficiency – if there is a need for rapid immunization or there is a risk that the patient will not report for subsequent visits. After the administration of a live vaccine, immunoglobulin preparations should not be administered for ≥2 weeks (this restriction does not apply to monoclonal antibody preparations) or blood products containing immunoglobulins, and if they were necessary, then it is worth considering repeating the vaccination after an appropriate period of time (3–11 months depending on the blood product and dose) or assessing the concentration of specific antibodies. Fortunately, the recommended additional vaccinations for asthma contain killed microorganisms or their fragments and are not subject to contraindications for live vaccines [31, 32].

Fortunately, the recommended additional vaccinations for asthma contain killed microorganisms or their fragments and do not share the contraindications that apply to live vaccines.

4.3 Special situations

Situations requiring special caution (i.e., considering with the patient whether the benefits of vaccination outweigh the risk of possible side effects or possibly modifying the vaccination schedule or technique (formerly relative or temporary contraindications)) are an acute disease with a severe or moderately severe course (including high fever; a mild disease, e.g., a cold, is not a contraindication to vaccination); exacerbation of chronic disease (until the symptoms of exacerbation subside and the patient's condition stabilizes); anaphylactic shock in the history (after another vaccine or a substance not included in the vaccine) – the risk of a systemic anaphylactic reaction (including shock) after vaccination may be higher than average in such people [31, 32].

Each of the vaccine components may cause a systemic (rarely, e.g., egg white or neomycin) or local (more often, e.g., thimerosal and aluminum) allergic reaction in an allergic person. The stoppers of vials or elements of pre-filled syringes of some preparations (made of dry natural rubber) contain latex which is dangerous for people allergic to this substance. Synthetic rubber, on the other hand, is completely safe from an allergological point of view. Before vaccination, carefully read the information provided in the manufacturer's leaflet and avoid preparations containing substances that the patient has not tolerated in the past (especially if they caused an anaphylactic reaction) or vaccines that are contraindicated in the patient [33].

Patients treated chronically with high doses of glucocorticosteroids may have a weakened immune response – in such cases, vaccinations should be planned appropriately in advance or performed after reducing the dose of glucocorticosteroids.

A significant problem that creates doubts about vaccinations may be biological treatment, allergen-specific immunotherapy (AIT) in patients with allergic asthma, or chronic use of immunoglobulin preparations in patients with certain immunodeficiencies. The vaccinations recommended for patients are inactivated vaccines; therefore, there is no need to maintain any time intervals between the administration of a biological drug or immunoglobulin preparations and the vaccination. Although there are no recommendations, it seems reasonable not to vaccinate the patient on the day of administration and 3–5 days before the administration of these drugs so that any adverse post-vaccination reactions are not confused with adverse drug reactions. There is a possibility of interactions between AIT preparations and vaccines against infectious diseases. In the case of subcutaneous immunotherapy (SCIT), a break of ≥7 days should be maintained between the protective vaccination and the administration of the allergen vaccine. There are no guidelines regarding protective vaccinations during sublingual immunotherapy (SLIT), although a break of several days is usually assumed in the case of vaccination in accordance with the Protective Vaccination Program. According to European Academy of Allergy and Clinical Immunology (EAACI) guidelines, COVID-19 vaccines should be administered like other vaccines, that is, 7 days after SCIT, and in the case of SLIT, the daily dose should be discontinued 3 days before COVID-19 vaccination and resumed 7 days later [34].

When discussing the issue of vaccinations, one cannot ignore the issue of adverse vaccine reactions (AVRs), which are disorders of health as a result of vaccination occurring within 4 weeks after the administration of the vaccine (or a longer period after vaccination against tuberculosis) resulting from a manufacturing defect of the preparation or a technical error during vaccination, or from the individual reaction of the patient to the vaccine. A serious AVR is considered to be death or life-threatening, a condition requiring or prolonging hospitalization, or permanent damage to health. A serious AVR is a reaction of particularly high intensity but does not require hospitalization and is not life-threatening. Fortunately, in most cases of health disorders after vaccination (suspected AVR), the relationship is coincidental (temporal coincidence) and not causal. Remember that in order to reduce the risk of AVRs, the patient should not perform intense physical activity, drink alcohol, or take painkillers from the non-steroidal anti-inflammatory drug group (NSAIDs) on the day of vaccination, as these factors may act as co-factors and trigger an allergic reaction [35].

5. Comprehensive therapeutic approach

A comprehensive therapeutic approach to asthma and immunodeficiencies focuses on effective treatment modification that takes into account the individual needs of patients. It includes both drug modification strategies and infection prevention, which is key to improving the quality of life of patients. Practical recommendations for therapy, including the role of vaccinations and health monitoring, are essential to provide effective care and optimize treatment outcomes.

An integrated approach to managing the health of patients with asthma and concomitant immunodeficiencies should primarily include:

- systematic patient education
- optimal asthma treatment with inhaled drugs
- patient diet and assessment of nutritional status (also in terms of non-nutritional immunomodulatory components)

- optimal treatment of concomitant diseases
- prevention of infections by avoiding contact with pathogens, additional vaccinations, and, in selected cases, post-exposure, temporary or chronic antimicrobial drug prophylaxis

Infection prevention in patients with asthma and immunodeficiencies is the foundation for preventing disease exacerbations and reducing the risk of hospitalization. It is important to educate patients about protection against microorganisms, including proper disinfection of hands and rooms, avoiding contact with infected people, and wearing protective masks.

Some patients require treatment with immunoglobulins. Due to the longest half-life, which is an average of 23 days, IgG antibodies are transfused. Indications for their use include deficiencies with reduced concentration of total IgG or IgG subclasses and specific antibody deficiency (SPAD), sometimes accompanied by acute autoimmune diseases. The degree of IgG concentration reduction does not determine the initiation of treatment, but it depends on the clinical condition of the patient. A practical scheme of the need to start immunoglobulin therapy is presented in **Figure 1**. The recommended initial dose of IgG replacement therapy is 400–600 mg/kg/4 weeks for the intravenous form and 100–150 mg/kg/week for the subcutaneous form. Remember that immunoglobulins are prepared from a pool of plasma from at least 1000 donors. In patients receiving these preparations, by determining antibodies in the IgG class (e.g., anti-HCV and antinuclear antibodies – ANA), we determine the antibodies of immunoglobulin donors. Diagnostics are reliable only after 4–6 weeks from discontinuing the preparation, of course, if there is no disorder in the production of antibodies in this class [37]. Currently, we have the possibility of intravenous or subcutaneous administration. Immunoglobulin replacement therapy is an effective tool in reducing the risk of respiratory infections in patients with

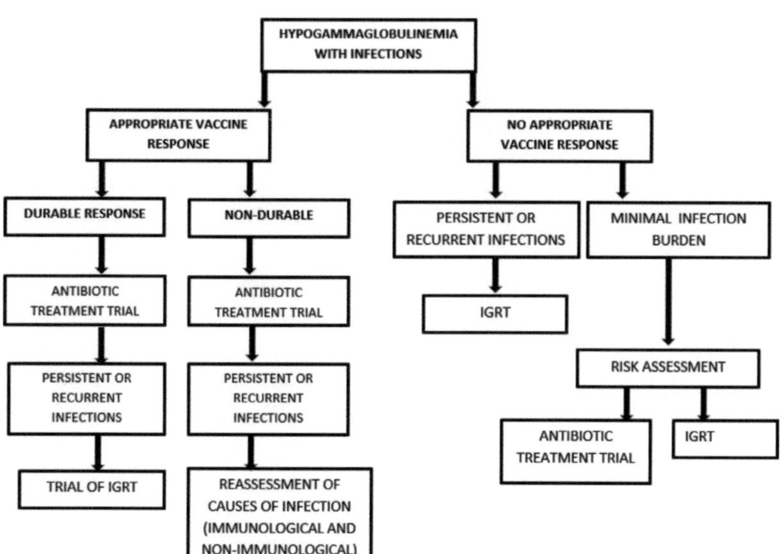

Figure 1.
Algorithm for assessing the indications for starting immunoglobulin replacement therapy (IGRT) [36].

hypogammaglobulinemia. Studies indicate that regular administration of immunoglobulins reduces the number of hospitalizations due to infections by as much as 50% while improving asthma control and reducing the need for corticosteroids [38]. However, the implementation of this therapy requires monitoring immunoglobulin concentrations to adjust its intensity to the individual needs of the patient.

An important aspect is the need for chronic antibiotic prophylaxis in some patients. Standard antibiotic regimens are derived primarily from data from immunocompetent patients with recurrent upper respiratory tract infections. Prophylaxis is usually initiated with amoxicillin, trimethoprim-sulfamethoxazole, or azithromycin. If these are ineffective, other agents such as amoxicillin-clavulanic acid or clarithromycin (or others) may be used. Some clinicians use full therapeutic doses, while others use half doses. In some centers, patients are rotated every 1–6 months, while in others, a single agent is continued. There are no published data on the efficacy of any specific regimen in this patient population. However, recent studies have focused on the use of azithromycin and have shown that its long-term prophylactic use in patients with primary antibody deficiencies (at least 3 times a week, for 3 consecutive days, in the former therapeutic dose or at half the dose), with coexisting chronic lung disease (including asthma, bronchiectasis) and recurrent/chronic respiratory tract infections is safe, reduces the frequency of exacerbations of lung disease, the frequency of additional antibiotic treatments and the number of hospitalizations, and improves the quality of life of patients. No increased drug resistance has been noted [39, 40].

The use of bacterial lysates, also known as "oral vaccines," requires clarification. Bacterial lysates are immunostimulatory agents derived from inactivated and lysed bacterial species. They are used in both prophylactic and therapeutic contexts to reduce the frequency and severity of recurrent respiratory tract infections. It should be remembered that they are contraindicated in acute infectious diseases, autoimmune diseases, immunosuppressive therapy, as well as in congenital and acquired immune disorders [41].

6. Summary

Asthma, as a chronic inflammatory disease of the airways, may be significantly influenced by both primary and secondary immunodeficiencies, which increase the risk of infections, exacerbate symptoms, and complicate treatment. This chapter highlights the importance of systematic diagnostic evaluation for immunodeficiencies in asthma patients, particularly those with severe or recurrent infections. It presents practical diagnostic algorithms, the most frequent types of immune defects, and their clinical features. The chapter also emphasizes the key role of vaccinations in the prevention of infections and asthma exacerbations, considering their safety and effectiveness in immunocompromised individuals. Special attention was given to therapy with immunoglobulins and long-term antibiotic prophylaxis in selected patients. A multidisciplinary, individualized, and preventive care strategy is essential for improving clinical outcomes and quality of life in asthma patients with immune disorders.

Author details

Katarzyna Napiórkowska-Baran
Department of Allergology, Clinical Immunology and Internal Diseases, Collegium Medicum Bydgoszcz, Nicolaus Copernicus University Toruń, Bydgoszcz, Poland

*Address all correspondence to: knapiorkowska@cm.umk.pl

References

[1] International Union of Immunological Societies. Human Inborn Errors of Immunity: 2024 Update on the Classification from the International Union of Immunological Societies Expert Committee. 2024. Available from: https://wp-iuis.s3.eu-west-1.amazonaws.com/app/uploads/2025/01/08170257/IEI-Final-Update-of-2024-Report-Jan-2025.pdf [Accessed: March 23, 2025]

[2] Ochs HD, Hagin D. Primary immunodeficiency disorders: General classification, new molecular insights, and practical approach to diagnosis and treatment. Annals of Allergy, Asthma & Immunology. 2014;**112**(6):489-495. DOI: 10.1016/j.anai.2014.04.007

[3] Jefrey Modell Foundation. Primary Immunodefciency Resource Centre. Available from: http://www.info4pi.org/library/educational-materials/10-warning-signs [Accessed: March 30, 2025]

[4] Kim VHD, Upton JEM, Derfalvi B, Hildebrand KJ, McCusker C. Inborn errors of immunity (primary immunodeficiencies). Allergy, Asthma and Clinical Immunology. 2025;**20**(Suppl. 3):76. DOI: 10.1186/s13223-024-00938-z

[5] Nguyen AT, Aquino MR. Primary antibody deficiencies. Allergy and Asthma Proceedings. 2024;**45**(5):310-316. DOI: 10.2500/aap.2024.45.240052

[6] Devonshire AL, Makhija M. Approach to primary immunodeficiency. Allergy and Asthma Proceedings. 2019;**40**(6):465-469. DOI: 10.2500/aap.2019.40.4273

[7] Bucciol G, Delafontaine S, Meyts I, Poli C. Inborn errors of immunity: A field without frontiers. Immunological Reviews. 2024;**322**(1):15-27. DOI: 10.1111/imr.13297

[8] El-Sayed ZA, El-Ghoneimy DH, Ortega-Martell JA, Radwan N, Aldave JC, Al-Herz W, et al. Allergic manifestations of inborn errors of immunity and their impact on the diagnosis: A worldwide study. World Allergy Organization Journal. 2022;**15**(6):100657. DOI: 10.1016/j.waojou.2022.100657

[9] Lee SH, Ban GY, Kim SC, Chung CG, Lee HY, Lee JH, et al. Association between primary immunodeficiency and asthma exacerbation in adult asthmatics. The Korean Journal of Internal Medicine. 2020;**35**(2):449-456. DOI: 10.3904/kjim.2018.413

[10] Delafontaine S, Meyts I. Infection and autoinflammation in inborn errors of immunity: Brothers in arms. Current Opinion in Immunology. 2021;**72**:331-339. DOI: 10.1016/j.coi.2021.08.004

[11] Napiórkowska-Baran K, Darwish S, Kaczor J, Treichel P, Szymczak B, Szota M, et al. Oral diseases as a manifestation of inborn errors of immunity. Journal of Clinical Medicine. 2024;**13**(17):5079. DOI: 10.3390/jcm13175079

[12] Napiórkowska-Baran K, Doligalska A, Drozd M, Czarnowska M, Łaszczych D, Dolina M, et al. Management of a Patient with cardiovascular disease should include assessment of primary and secondary Immunodeficiencies: Part 2-secondary Immunodeficiencies. Healthcare (Basel). 2024;**12**(19):1977. DOI: 10.3390/healthcare12191977

[13] Tuano KS, Seth N, Chinen J. Secondary immunodeficiencies: An overview. Annals of Allergy, Asthma

and Immunology. 2021;**127**(6):617-626. DOI: 10.1016/j.anai.2021.08.413

[14] Herman KE, Tuttle KL. Overview of secondary immunodeficiency. Allergy and Asthma Proceedings. 2024;**45**(5):347-354. DOI: 10.2500/aap.2024.45.240063

[15] Oghbaei M, Prakash J. Effect of primary processing of cereals and legumes on its nutritional quality: A comprehensive review. Cogent Food and Agriculture. 2016;**2**(1):1-14. DOI: 10.1080/23311932.2015.1136015

[16] Whitfield KC, Smith TJ, Rohner F, Wieringa FT, Green TJ. Thiamine fortification strategies in low- and middle-income settings: A review. Annals of the New York Academy of Sciences. 2021;**1498**(1):29-45. DOI: 10.1111/nyas.14565

[17] Mayer AB, Trenchard L, Rayns F. Historical changes in the mineral content of fruit and vegetables in the UK from 1940 to 2019: A concern for human nutrition and agriculture. International Journal of Food Sciences and Nutrition. 2022;**73**(3):315-326. DOI: 10.1080/09637486.2021.1981831

[18] Erisman JW. Nature-based agriculture for an adequate human microbiome. Organic Agriculture. 2021;**11**:225-230. DOI: 10.1007/s13165-020-00304-4

[19] Jartti T, Bønnelykke K, Elenius V, Feleszko W. Role of viruses in asthma. Seminars in Immunopathology. 2020;**42**(1):61-74. DOI: 10.1007/s00281-020-00781-5

[20] Anderson GP. Prospects for an asthma vaccine. Respirology. 2010;**15**(6):902-908. DOI: 10.1111/j.1440-1843.2010.01820.x

[21] Balzar S, Strand M, Nakano T, Wenzel SE. Subtle immunodeficiency in severe asthma: IgA and IgG2 correlate with lung function and symptoms. International Archives of Allergy and Immunology. 2006;**140**(2):96-102. DOI: 10.1159/000092252

[22] Monahan R, Otani IM, Lehman HK, Mustafa SS. A second look at secondary hypogammaglobulinemia. Annals of Allergy, Asthma and Immunology. 2025;**134**(3):269-278. DOI: 10.1016/j.anai.2024.12.003

[23] Perry TT, Grant TL, Dantzer JA, Udemgba C, Jefferson AA. Impact of socioeconomic factors on allergic diseases. The Journal of Allergy and Clinical Immunology. 2024;**153**(2):368-377. DOI: 10.1016/j.jaci.2023.10.025

[24] Bousquet J, Bousquet PJ, Godard P, Daures JP. The public health implications of asthma. Bulletin of the World Health Organization. 2005;**83**(7):548-554

[25] Sobh A, Bonilla FA. Vaccination in primary immunodeficiency disorders. The Journal of Allergy and Clinical Immunology. In Practice. 2016;**4**(6):1066-1075. DOI: 10.1016/j.jaip.2016.09.012

[26] Farrar JL, Childs L, Ouattara M, Akhter F, Britton A, Pilishvili T, et al. Systematic review and meta-analysis of the efficacy and effectiveness of pneumococcal vaccines in adults. Pathogens. 2023;**12**(5):732. DOI: 10.3390/pathogens12050732

[27] Safonova E, Yawn BP, Welte T, Wang C. Risk factors for herpes zoster: Should people with asthma or COPD be vaccinated? Respiratory Research. 2023;**24**(1):35. DOI: 10.1186/s12931-022-02305-1

[28] Wagner A, Weinberger B. Vaccines to prevent infectious diseases in the older population: Immunological challenges and future perspectives. Frontiers in

Immunology. 2020;**11**:717. DOI: 10.3389/fimmu.2020.00717

[29] Lee ARYB, Wong SY, Chai LYA, Lee SC, Lee MX, Muthiah MD, et al. Efficacy of covid-19 vaccines in immunocompromised patients: Systematic review and meta-analysis. BMJ. 2022;**376**:e068632. DOI: 10.1136/bmj-2021-068632

[30] Pöyhönen L, Bustamante J, Casanova JL, Jouanguy E, Zhang Q. Life-threatening infections due to live-attenuated vaccines: Early manifestations of inborn errors of immunity. Journal of Clinical Immunology. 2019;**39**(4):376-390. DOI: 10.1007/s10875-019-00642-3. Epub 2019 May 23. Erratum in: J Clin Immunol. 2019;39(5):527. doi: 10.1007/s10875-019-00653-0

[31] Opri R, Zanoni G, Caffarelli C, Bottau P, Caimmi S, Crisafulli G, et al. True and false contraindications to vaccines. Allergol Immunopathol (Madr). 2018;**46**(1):99-104. DOI: 10.1016/j.aller.2017.02.003

[32] Smith M. Vaccine safety: Medical contraindications, myths, and risk communication. Pediatrics in Review. 2015;**36**(6):227-238. DOI: 10.1542/pir.36-6-227. Erratum in: Pediatr Rev. 2015 Aug;36(8):369. doi: 10.1542/pir.36-8-369

[33] Aytekin ES, Şekerel BE, Şahiner ÜM. Allergic reactions during childhood vaccination and management. The Turkish Journal of Pediatrics. 2021;**63**(6):941-954. DOI: 10.24953/turkjped.2021.06.001

[34] Nilsson L, Brockow K, Alm J, Cardona V, Caubet JC, Gomes E, et al. Vaccination and allergy: EAACI position paper, practical aspects. Pediatric Allergy and Immunology. 2017;**28**(7):628-640. DOI: 10.1111/pai.12762

[35] Des Roches A, Graham F, Begin P, Paradis L, Gold M. Evaluation of adverse reactions to vaccines. The Journal of Allergy and Clinical Immunology. In Practice. 2021;**9**(10):3584-3597. DOI: 10.1016/j.jaip.2021.08.002

[36] Jolles S, Chapel H, Litzman J. When to initiate immunoglobulin replacement therapy (IGRT) in antibody deficiency: A practical approach. Clinical and Experimental Immunology. 2017;**188**(3):333-341. DOI: 10.1111/cei.12915

[37] Wasserman RL. Personalized therapy: Immunoglobulin replacement for antibody deficiency. Immunology and Allergy Clinics of North America. 2019;**39**(1):95-111. DOI: 10.1016/j.iac.2018.08.001

[38] Kim JH, Ye YM, Ban GY, Shin YS, Lee HY, Nam YH, et al. Effects of immunoglobulin replacement on asthma exacerbation in adult asthmatics with IgG subclass deficiency. Allergy, Asthma and Immunology Research. 2017;**9**(6):526-533. DOI: 10.4168/aair.2017.9.6.526

[39] Milito C, Pulvirenti F, Cinetto F, Lougaris V, Soresina A, Pecoraro A, et al. Double-blind, placebo-controlled, randomized trial on low-dose azithromycin prophylaxis in patients with primary antibody deficiencies. The Journal of Allergy and Clinical Immunology. 2019;**144**(2):584-593.e7. DOI: 10.1016/j.jaci.2019.01.051

[40] Kuruvilla M, de la Morena MT. Antibiotic prophylaxis in primary immune deficiency disorders. The Journal of Allergy and Clinical Immunology. In Practice. 2013;**1**(6):573-582. DOI: 10.1016/j.jaip.2013.09.013

[41] Jurkiewicz D, Zielnik-Jurkiewicz B. Bacterial lysates in the prevention of respiratory tract infections. Otolaryngologia Polska. 2018;**72**(5):1-8. DOI: 10.5604/01.3001.0012.7216

Chapter 4

Asthma as a Comorbidity in Primary Ciliary Dyskinesia: Pathophysiology and Therapeutic Approaches

Wilfredo De Jesús-Rojas, Gabriel Román-Ríos and Ricardo A. Mosquera

Abstract

Primary Ciliary Dyskinesia (PCD) is a rare genetic disorder resulting in impaired mucociliary clearance due to dysfunctional motile cilia. Patients commonly experience chronic respiratory symptoms, including persistent cough, recurrent infections, and bronchiectasis. Bronchial asthma, a highly prevalent airway disease characterized by airway obstruction and airway hyperreactivity, shares several clinical features with PCD, such as cough and shortness of breath. This overlap poses diagnostic and therapeutic challenges, particularly when features of both diseases coexist in the same patient. In recent years, asthma has emerged as a potential comorbidity in PCD, prompting interest in understanding the mechanistic and clinical intersections between these two conditions. This chapter explores the pathophysiological differences and similarities between asthma and PCD, focusing on distinct inflammatory pathways, ciliary function, and airway remodeling. Diagnostic strategies are discussed, with attention to the pitfalls of misclassification and the value of lung function, nitric oxide measurements, and genetic testing. Therapeutic implications are also examined, including the role of inhaled corticosteroids, bronchodilators, airway clearance techniques, and macrolide therapy in patients with dual pathology. By synthesizing current clinical insights and research findings, this chapter aims to guide clinicians in recognizing asthma as a comorbidity in PCD and applying tailored treatment approaches that address the complex respiratory needs of this unique patient population.

Keywords: primary ciliary dyskinesia, bronchial asthma, mucociliary clearance, airway inflammation, respiratory comorbidities

1. Introduction

Primary Ciliary Dyskinesia (PCD) is a rare, genetically inherited disorder characterized by abnormalities in the structure and function of motile cilia [1–3]. These microscopic, hair-like projections line the respiratory tract and are essential

IntechOpen

for mucociliary clearance, a defense mechanism that removes inhaled pathogens, allergens, and debris [4]. In individuals with PCD, defective ciliary motility leads to impaired airway clearance, resulting in chronic respiratory infections, persistent wet cough, sinusitis, otitis media, and progressive bronchiectasis [4, 5]. The disease is typically diagnosed in childhood but is often underrecognized due to overlapping symptoms with other respiratory conditions, including asthma [1, 6].

Asthma is one of the most common chronic diseases worldwide, affecting over 300 million individuals [7]. It is characterized by variable airflow obstruction, airway hyperresponsiveness, and chronic inflammation, often driven by Th2-mediated immune responses [8–11]. Asthma presents with symptoms such as wheezing, coughing, chest tightness, and shortness of breath and can range from mild to life-threatening [9, 12]. Despite the availability of effective treatments, asthma continues to impose a significant burden on healthcare systems due to frequent exacerbations, hospitalizations, and impaired quality of life [13].

The clinical similarities between PCD and asthma—including shared symptoms like shortness of breath and cough—can complicate diagnosis and management [14]. Furthermore, recent studies have identified a subset of patients with PCD who also meet diagnostic criteria for asthma, raising important questions about comorbidity, overlapping pathophysiology, and implications for treatment [1]. Exploring asthma as a comorbidity in PCD is essential for accurate diagnosis, personalized treatment strategies, and improved outcomes [14].

This chapter aims to (1) review the pathophysiological basis of both diseases, (2) discuss their clinical and diagnostic overlap, (3) examine therapeutic challenges, and (4) provide evidence-informed approaches for managing patients with both PCD and asthma.

2. Primary ciliary dyskinesia: Clinical and genetic overview

PCD is a rare genetic disorder, most commonly inherited in an autosomal recessive pattern, though X-linked inheritance has also been documented [1–3, 15]. It affects the structure and function of motile cilia, which play a critical role in mucociliary clearance in the respiratory tract, as well as in embryonic development and reproductive function [16]. Pathogenic genetic variants in genes responsible for ciliary components disrupt coordinated ciliary beating, leading to impaired mucus clearance and resulting in recurrent and chronic respiratory infections [17].

The ultrastructure of normal motile cilia is highly conserved and critical for their function [18]. In cross-section, a healthy cilium displays a characteristic "9+2" axonemal arrangement, consisting of nine outer microtubule doublets surrounding a central pair of singlet microtubules [16, 18]. Anchored to each outer doublet are outer and inner dynein arms—motor proteins responsible for generating the sliding motion that drives coordinated ciliary beating. Additional structural elements, such as radial spokes and nexin links, provide stability and regulate the waveform [16, 18, 19]. At the base of each cilium lies the basal body, which serves as the nucleation point and anchoring structure [20].

In PCD, genetic variants in genes encoding for more than 200 structural proteins result in ciliary ultrastructural abnormalities that impair motility [21]. One common defect is the absence of the central pair of microtubules, producing a "9+0" pattern rather than the normal 9+2 configuration [22]. This is typically observed in patients with pathogenic genetic variants in *RSPH1*, *RSPH4A*, or *RSPH9*, which are associated with central apparatus (CA) defects [22]. As illustrated in **Figure 1**, this central pair defect disrupts the cilium's ability to perform its regular, coordinated beating pattern, leading to rotational, or dyskinetic cilia [23]. Such structural defects directly compromise mucociliary clearance, setting the stage for chronic infections, bronchiectasis, and other complications of PCD [17, 24].

2.1 Genetic basis and common genetic variants

Over 55 genes have been implicated in PCD, many of which encode components of the ciliary axoneme, such as dynein arms, radial spokes, and central pair structures. One of the most well-characterized genetic variants in specific populations is the *RSPH4A* founder variant, particularly prevalent in Puerto Rico [25–27]. This genetic variant affects the radial spoke head protein 4A, contributing to central pair defects and abnormal ciliary motion [25, 26, 28]. Other commonly affected genes include *DNAH5, DNAI1, CCDC39*, and *CCDC40*, among others [24]. Genetic variants vary by population, and whole-exome sequencing has become an essential tool in identifying new causative variants [29].

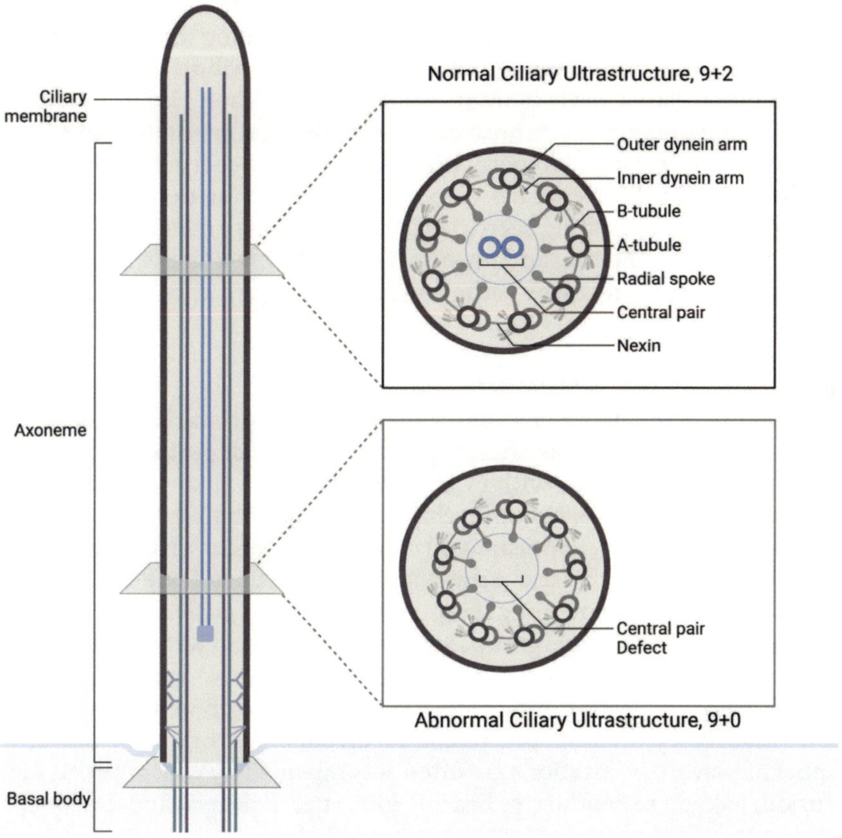

Figure 1.
Ultrastructural comparison of normal and PCD-affected motile cilia. Schematic representation of the ultrastructure of a normal motile cilium (top) and a cilium with a central pair defect (bottom) commonly seen in Primary Ciliary Dyskinesia (PCD). The normal "9+2" arrangement features nine outer microtubule doublets and a central pair, while the PCD cilium lacks the central pair, forming a "9+0" configuration associated with impaired motility.

2.2 Pathophysiology of mucociliary dysfunction

The hallmark of PCD lies in the dysfunction of motile cilia, specialized organelles on the apical surface of epithelial cells that line the respiratory tract, paranasal sinuses, middle ear, and reproductive organs [20, 23]. In healthy individuals, motile cilia beat in a highly coordinated, wave-like pattern to drive the movement of the mucus layer along the airway surface [20]. This process, known as mucociliary clearance, is essential for the removal of inhaled particles, pathogens, and environmental debris from the respiratory tract [2, 20].

In PCD, structural defects in the ciliary axoneme—often involving dynein arms, radial spokes, or central pairs—result in abnormal, inefficient, or completely absent ciliary motion [30]. This leads to impaired mucociliary clearance, which has cascading effects on respiratory health [6]. Without effective clearance, mucus becomes stagnant in the airways, creating a favorable environment for bacterial colonization and persistent inflammation [31]. Over time, this leads to chronic infections, neutrophilic inflammation, tissue damage, and bronchiectasis [32].

Ultrastructural abnormalities observed in PCD vary depending on the underlying genetic variant. For example, the absence of outer dynein arms is commonly seen in *DNAH5* variants [33]. These defects are visible on transmission electron microscopy and increasingly through immunofluorescence-based staining for ciliary proteins [34]. The persistent accumulation of thick mucus also contributes to airway obstruction and atelectasis, particularly in infants and young children [35]. As the disease progresses, the inflammatory response becomes chronic, contributing to epithelial remodeling, submucosal gland hyperplasia, and irreversible structural damage [36]. **Figure 2** illustrates the difference between healthy ciliary function and the dysfunctional, ineffective ciliary beating seen in PCD. The contrast between efficient mucus transport in healthy epithelium and mucus stasis in PCD highlights the central role of ciliary dysfunction in the disease's pathogenesis.

2.3 Clinical manifestations

PCD is a multisystem disorder with hallmark features primarily affecting the respiratory tract [37]. Symptoms often begin in the neonatal period, where approximately 80–90% of term infants with PCD present with unexplained respiratory distress requiring oxygen support or mechanical ventilation [38]. This neonatal presentation may include tachypnea, nasal congestion, retractions, and lobar atelectasis—frequently mistaken for transient tachypnea or neonatal pneumonia [39].

As children grow, the respiratory symptoms persist and evolve. One of the most consistent features across all age groups is a daily, year-round wet (productive) cough, often misattributed to recurrent viral infections, recurrent bronchiolitis, or asthma [40]. Chronic nasal congestion and rhinorrhea typically begin in infancy and are frequently associated with nasal polyps and recurrent or chronic rhinosinusitis [41]. These upper airway manifestations are often accompanied by chronic otitis media with effusion, leading to conductive hearing loss, speech delays, and a frequent need for repeated placement of tympanostomy tubes [42, 43].

Lower airway disease in PCD progressively worsens, with repeated infections and inflammation eventually leading to bronchiectasis, most commonly in the middle and lower lobes [44]. This structural lung damage can result in impaired gas exchange and reduced exercise tolerance [45, 46]. Digital clubbing may be observed in older children or adults with advanced lung disease [47].

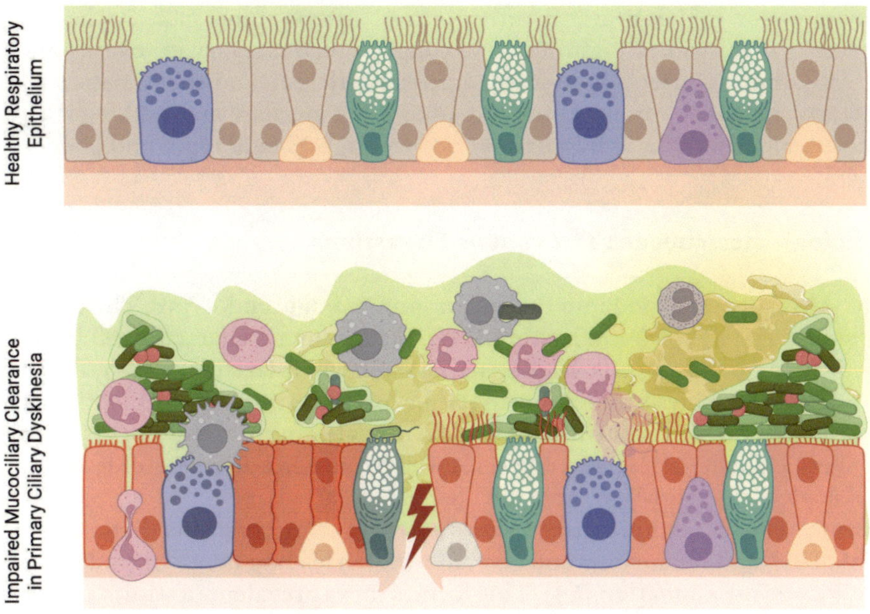

Figure 2.
Healthy versus dysfunctional airway epithelium in primary ciliary dyskinesia. Schematic comparison of healthy respiratory epithelium (upper panel) and the airway epithelium in Primary Ciliary Dyskinesia (PCD) (lower panel). In healthy tissue, motile cilia and coordinated mucus production maintain effective mucociliary clearance and protect the airway from pathogens. In PCD, ciliary dysfunction leads to impaired clearance, mucus accumulation, and microbial colonization. This environment promotes chronic neutrophilic inflammation, epithelial damage, and increased susceptibility to infection and airway remodeling.

A distinctive hallmark of PCD is the presence of laterality defects. Approximately 50% of patients exhibit situs inversus totalis (complete mirror-image reversal of thoracic and abdominal organs), which, when accompanied by bronchiectasis and chronic sinusitis, constitutes the classic triad known as Kartagener's Syndrome [48, 49]. More complex laterality defects, such as heterotaxy, congenital heart defects, and splenic anomalies, can also occur due to the role of motile cilia in embryonic left-right axis formation [50, 51].

Other manifestations may include male infertility due to impaired flagellar motility in spermatozoa and female subfertility related to dysfunction of fallopian tube cilia [52]. Gastrointestinal symptoms such as gastroesophageal reflux disease (GERD) are frequently reported, likely secondary to chronic coughing and altered intrathoracic pressure dynamics [53, 54].

The progression and severity of symptoms can vary widely among individuals, influenced by genotype, access to care, and comorbidities. Timely recognition of this characteristic constellation of signs—especially chronic wet cough and neonatal respiratory distress—can facilitate early referral for diagnostic testing and prompt initiation of appropriate interventions.

3. Bronchial asthma: Definition, endotypes, and phenotypes

Bronchial asthma is a chronic inflammatory disease of the airways characterized by variable and reversible airflow obstruction, bronchial hyperresponsiveness, and airway inflammation [55]. It presents with intermittent symptoms such as wheezing, shortness of breath, chest tightness, and cough, which can vary in severity and frequency [56]. Asthma affects individuals across the lifespan and encompasses a wide spectrum of clinical presentations and underlying mechanisms, making it a heterogeneous condition that is best understood through its endotypes and phenotypes [57, 58].

3.1 Immunologic mechanisms: Th2 vs. non-Th2 asthma

Asthma is broadly classified into two major immunologic endotypes: Th2 (Type 2-high) and non-Th2 (Type 2-low) asthma [59]. Th2 asthma is characterized by the activation of type 2 helper T cells, leading to the release of interleukins IL-4, IL-5, and IL-13 [60]. These cytokines promote eosinophilic inflammation, IgE production, and mucus hypersecretion [61]. This form of asthma often begins in childhood, is associated with allergic sensitization, and responds well to inhaled corticosteroids and targeted biologics (e.g., anti-IL-5, anti-IgE) [62, 63].

In contrast, non-Th2 asthma encompasses a variety of mechanisms that may include Th1, Th17, and innate immune responses, often leading to neutrophilic or paucigranulocytic inflammation [64]. This form is more prevalent in adults and may be triggered by infections, pollutants, or occupational exposures [64, 65]. Non-Th2 asthma tends to be more resistant to corticosteroid therapy and lacks well-defined biomarkers, posing therapeutic challenges [66, 67].

3.2 Inflammatory pathways and triggers

Asthma inflammation involves a cascade of immune cell recruitment, mediator release, and structural changes to the airways [68]. Common triggers include allergens, respiratory infections, air pollution, exercise, and cold air [69]. In Th2 asthma, eosinophils dominate the airway milieu, whereas in non-Th2 asthma, neutrophils or mixed cell infiltrates may predominate [70]. Chronic inflammation leads to airway remodeling, including subepithelial fibrosis, smooth muscle hypertrophy, and mucus gland hyperplasia, contributing to persistent airflow limitation in some patients [71, 72].

3.3 Diagnosis and misdiagnosis in children and adults

Diagnosing asthma involves a combination of clinical assessment, spirometry demonstrating reversible airflow obstruction, and evaluation of symptom variability [73]. In children, diagnosis can be particularly challenging due to overlapping symptoms with other respiratory conditions such as viral bronchiolitis, recurrent pulmonary infections, or, as seen in PCD, chronic productive cough [74]. In adults, late-onset asthma can mimic or overlap with chronic obstructive pulmonary disease (COPD) or other structural lung diseases [75].

Asthma is often misdiagnosed, with both overdiagnosis and underdiagnosis contributing to delayed treatment [76]. Some patients with chronic cough or wheeze may be labeled as asthmatic without objective testing, while others with atypical features (e.g., persistent wet cough, poor response to bronchodilators) may have alternative or coexisting conditions like PCD [76, 77]. Careful evaluation using lung function testing, biomarkers (e.g., FeNO, nNO), imaging, and, when appropriate, genetic testing is critical for accurate diagnosis and optimal management.

4. Overlap and diagnostic challenges between asthma and PCD

PCD and bronchial asthma are distinct respiratory disorders with differing pathophysiological mechanisms. However, they often present with overlapping clinical features, leading to diagnostic challenges [14].

4.1 Shared clinical features: Wheezing, cough, and airflow obstruction

Both PCD and asthma commonly manifest with symptoms such as chronic cough and airflow limitation [78, 79]. In asthma, these symptoms result from airway inflammation and hyperresponsiveness, leading to reversible bronchoconstriction [80]. Conversely, in PCD, defective motile cilia impair mucociliary clearance, resulting in mucus stasis, recurrent infections, and chronic inflammation [81]. This can lead to airway obstruction and bronchiectasis, mimicking asthma symptoms [82]. Clinical similarities can lead to misdiagnosis, particularly when comprehensive diagnostic evaluations—such as those conducted at a specialized PCD center—are limited in multiple countries [83]. **Figure 3** depicts overlapping symptoms of PCD and bronchial asthma.

4.1.1 Characteristic symptoms of PCD

- *Neonatal respiratory distress*: Breathing difficulties in full-term newborns
- *Chronic wet cough*: Persistent, productive cough starting in early childhood
- *Chronic nasal congestion and sinusitis*: Persistent nasal blockage and sinus infections
- *Recurrent otitis media*: Frequent middle ear infections leading to potential hearing loss

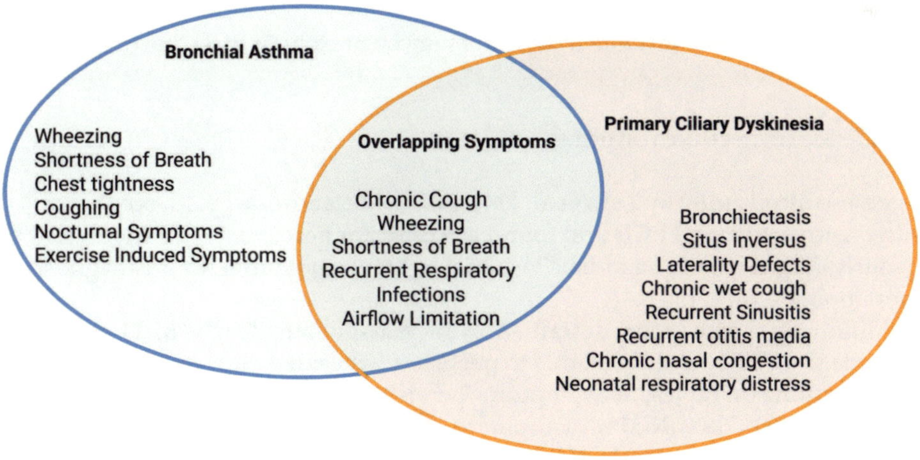

Figure 3.
Venn diagram showing the distinct and overlapping symptoms of Primary Ciliary Dyskinesia (PCD) and bronchial asthma. Characteristic asthma symptoms include chest tightness and nocturnal and exercise-induced symptoms. Characteristic PCD features include neonatal respiratory distress, chronic wet cough, and laterality defects. Shared symptoms such as chronic cough, wheezing, and shortness of breath may lead to diagnostic challenges.

- *Bronchiectasis*: Structural enlargement of the bronchi or bronchioles
- *Situs inversus/laterality defects*: Mirror-image reversal of internal organs in approximately 50% of cases

4.1.2 Characteristic symptoms of asthma

- *Wheezing*: A whistling sound when breathing, especially during exhalation
- *Shortness of breath*: Difficulty breathing or feeling out of breath
- *Chest tightness*: A feeling of pressure or constriction in the chest
- *Coughing*: Often worse at night or early morning; may be dry or productive with clear or white secretions
- *Exercise-induced symptoms*: Symptoms triggered or worsened by physical activity
- *Nocturnal symptoms*: Symptoms that worsen at night, potentially disrupting sleep

4.1.3 Overlapping symptoms between PCD and asthma

- *Chronic cough*: Persistent coughing present in both conditions
- *Wheezing*: Common in asthma; may occur in PCD due to mucus obstruction
- *Shortness of breath*: Experienced during asthma attacks and episodes of infection-associated bronchiectasis in PCD
- *Recurrent respiratory infections*: Frequent lung infections seen in both conditions
- *Airflow limitation*: Variable in asthma; may be present in PCD due to mucus buildup

4.2 Evidence from clinical studies

A case-control study by Zein et al. [14] analyzed electronic health records of children with confirmed PCD and found a significant percentage of patients had been previously diagnosed with asthma. This highlights the potential for misdiagnosis due to overlapping symptoms [14].

Additionally, a case report described an 18-year-old female who had been treated for asthma since early childhood due to persistent wheezing and cough. Despite standard asthma therapies, her symptoms persisted. Further investigations, including nasal Nitric Oxide (nNO) measurement and electron microscopy of nasal cilia, confirmed a diagnosis of PCD [84].

4.3 Importance of considering PCD in nonresponsive asthma cases

In patients with asthma-like symptoms unresponsive to standard therapies, especially those with persistent wet cough, chronic sinusitis, or otitis media, clinicians should consider alternative diagnoses such as PCD [85]. Diagnostic evaluations for PCD include nNO measurement, high-speed video microscopy of ciliary motion, electron microscopy of ciliary ultrastructure, and genetic testing [28, 86, 87]. Early and accurate diagnosis is crucial for implementing appropriate management strategies, including airway clearance therapies and targeted antibiotic treatments, which differ significantly from standard asthma management [88]. Recognizing the potential overlap between asthma and PCD is essential to avoid misdiagnosis and ensure patients receive appropriate and effective care tailored to their specific condition.

5. Epidemiology of asthma in PCD patients

Understanding the epidemiology of asthma among individuals with PCD is essential for both clinical management and diagnostic precision. Although the two diseases are pathophysiologically distinct, recent evidence has revealed an increasing recognition of bronchial asthma features, including reversible airway obstruction, in patients with genetically confirmed PCD [89].

5.1 Prevalence of reversible airway obstruction in PCD

Traditionally, asthma has been excluded from the PCD phenotype due to the neutrophilic, non-Th2 nature of inflammation observed in PCD airways. However, studies such as Levine et al. [89] have challenged this notion. In their retrospective analysis of spirometry data from PCD patients, over 50% demonstrated bronchodilator responsiveness, a hallmark of asthma. These findings suggest that reversible airway obstruction may be more prevalent in PCD than previously appreciated, raising the possibility of a true overlap phenotype or at least shared functional consequences in the airways.

5.2 Data from registries and case series

Large PCD registries, including the international PCD (iPCD) cohort and national databases, have begun capturing data on asthma diagnoses and bronchodilator use in patients with PCD [90]. These data reveal that asthma is often recorded as a comorbidity or even as an initial diagnosis before PCD is confirmed [90]. Case series have similarly reported individuals initially treated for asthma who were later diagnosed with PCD, particularly in settings where chronic wet cough and recurrent infections were initially attributed to poorly controlled asthma [91–93]. The lack of early suspicion for PCD contributes to diagnostic delays and suboptimal treatment in many patients [94].

5.3 Phenotypic overlap and under-recognition

The clinical overlap between asthma and PCD includes chronic cough and reduced lung function [95]. However, the underlying mechanisms differ: asthma is driven by Th2-mediated eosinophilic inflammation [96], while PCD features a neutrophil-dominated profile due to persistent infection and mucus stasis [97]. Despite these distinctions, the frequent use of asthma-related terminology and treatments in PCD patients highlights a pattern of under-recognition. Particularly in children, where wheezing is a nonspecific finding, the potential for misdiagnosis is high. Without access to specialized diagnostic tools—such as nNO testing, high-speed video microscopy, or genetic sequencing—many cases of PCD are mislabeled as atypical or treatment-resistant asthma with high doses of inhaled corticosteroids [98].

As research expands and registries grow, a clearer epidemiological profile is emerging. It suggests that asthma-like features are not uncommon in PCD, either as misdiagnosed symptoms or as a genuine comorbidity. Further investigation is needed to define clinical subgroups, understand shared inflammatory pathways, and develop tailored therapeutic approaches for patients with features of both diseases.

6. Pathophysiological intersections between asthma and primary ciliary dyskinesia

Although asthma and PCD are distinct conditions, they share intersecting features in their impact on airway function and inflammation. Understanding the differences and points of convergence in their underlying pathophysiology is critical to avoid misdiagnosis and guide appropriate therapeutic decisions, especially in patients with overlapping clinical features.

6.1 Mucociliary clearance impairment and antigen retention

One of the central features of PCD is defective mucociliary clearance due to structural or functional abnormalities in motile cilia [99]. In healthy airways, cilia propel mucus and entrapped particles toward the oropharynx, protecting the lungs from infection and inflammation [100]. In PCD, impaired ciliary motion leads to mucus stasis, bacterial colonization, and chronic infection [101]. This stagnation of secretions also results in prolonged antigen exposure and retention in the airways [102].

Interestingly, a similar downstream effect may occur in some forms of severe or poorly controlled asthma. In particular, airway remodeling, mucus plugging, and epithelial barrier disruption in chronic asthma may impair local clearance mechanisms, enhancing antigen persistence and driving further immune activation [103]. However, in asthma, the dysfunction is not due to ciliary defects but rather secondary to inflammation and structural changes [104].

6.2 Neutrophilic vs. eosinophilic inflammation

The dominant inflammatory phenotype in PCD is neutrophilic, driven by chronic bacterial infections like *Pseudomonas aeruginosa* and innate immune activation [105]. This leads to persistent neutrophil infiltration in the airways, elevated levels of neutrophil elastase, and progressive tissue damage [106, 107].

In contrast, eosinophilic inflammation is the hallmark of type 2 (Th2)-high asthma, where cytokines like IL-5 and IL-13 promote eosinophil recruitment, mucus hypersecretion, and IgE production [108]. However, some patients with asthma—particularly those with adult-onset, obesity-related, or severe phenotypes—exhibit neutrophilic or mixed granulocytic inflammation, resembling the airway profile seen in PCD [109].

The overlap in inflammatory patterns, especially in steroid-resistant asthma and in PCD patients with reversible airway obstruction, has sparked interest in exploring shared pathways and tailored treatments based on specific endotypes rather than a one-size-fits-all approach.

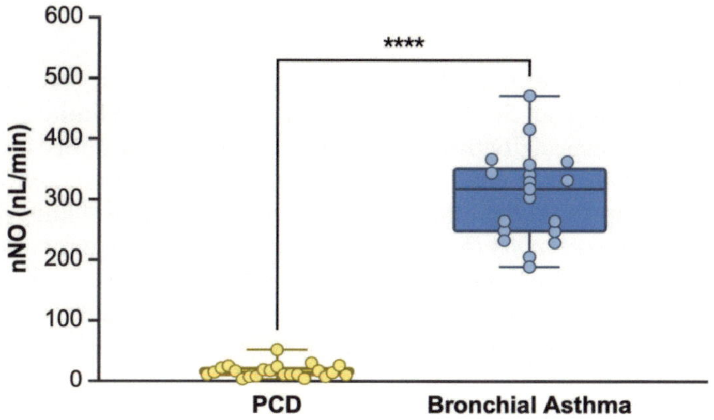

Figure 4.
Nasal nitric oxide (nNO) levels in primary ciliary dyskinesia (PCD) and bronchial asthma. Box-and-whisker plot comparing nasal nitric oxide (nNO) levels between individuals with PCD and those with bronchial asthma. PCD patients exhibit significantly reduced nNO concentrations, typically below 77 nL/min, consistent with impaired ciliary function. In contrast, asthma patients demonstrate elevated nNO levels due to airway inflammation. This biomarker serves as a useful diagnostic tool to differentiate between the two conditions.

6.3 Role of nitric oxide in asthma and PCD

The nNO serves as a useful biomarker in differentiating asthma from PCD [110, 111]. In PCD, nNO levels are characteristically low, often less than 77 nL/min when measured by chemiluminescence, due to defective production or release from paranasal sinus epithelium [87, 112]. This low level is a diagnostic clue and has been incorporated into screening algorithms for suspected PCD (**Figure 4**) [112].

Conversely, patients with asthma—especially those with type 2 inflammation—typically have elevated exhaled nitric oxide (FeNO) levels, reflecting increased inducible nitric oxide synthase (iNOS) activity in inflamed epithelial cells [113]. This elevation correlates with eosinophilic airway inflammation and is used clinically to support asthma diagnosis, monitor treatment response, and guide corticosteroid use [114].

These divergent nitric oxide profiles highlight the contrasting mechanisms underlying airway inflammation and serve as important biomarkers to distinguish PCD from asthma when clinical features overlap.

Understanding these pathophysiological intersections supports a more nuanced view of respiratory disease and encourages clinicians to move beyond symptom-based diagnoses to integrate molecular, inflammatory, and functional markers in their diagnostic and therapeutic strategies.

7. Therapeutic considerations in the management of PCD with asthma-like features

Managing respiratory symptoms in patients with PCD requires a detailed approach, particularly when asthma-like features such as wheezing or reversible airway obstruction are present. Treatment must be tailored to address both the underlying defect in mucociliary clearance and any coexisting airway hyperresponsiveness or inflammation.

7.1 Inhaled corticosteroids and bronchodilators in PCD

While inhaled corticosteroids (ICS) are the cornerstone of asthma management, their role in PCD is less clear. Studies suggest that ICS may have limited benefit in typical PCD patients, especially those without eosinophilic inflammation [115]. However, in cases where bronchial hyperreactivity or true asthma coexist with PCD, ICS may provide symptom relief and reduce inflammation [116]. Similarly, short-acting or long-acting beta-agonists (SABA/LABA) may be useful in patients demonstrating bronchodilator responsiveness on spirometry [117, 118]. A trial of bronchodilator therapy may be appropriate for PCD patients with documented airway reversibility, but the response should be monitored closely to avoid overtreatment [89].

7.2 Role of airway clearance and physiotherapy

Airway clearance remains the cornerstone of PCD management [118]. Daily physiotherapy techniques such as chest percussion, positive expiratory pressure (PEP) devices, autogenic drainage, and high-frequency chest wall oscillation are critical to mobilize mucus and prevent infection [119]. Inhaled hypertonic saline may be added to enhance secretion clearance [120]. Unlike asthma, where airway clearance is not routinely emphasized, in PCD it is foundational and should be prioritized in all patients [121].

7.3 Macrolides and anti-inflammatory therapies

Chronic macrolide therapy (e.g., azithromycin) has gained interest in PCD due to its combined antimicrobial and immunomodulatory effects. Studies have shown that long-term macrolide use can reduce the frequency of exacerbations and improve quality of life in PCD patients [122, 123]. Macrolides are particularly beneficial in individuals with frequent bacterial colonization or those who experience neutrophilic-driven inflammation [124]. While they are not part of standard asthma management, their use in PCD may address both the infectious colonization and inflammatory components of the disease [125].

7.4 Personalized approaches based on phenotype

Given the heterogeneity of both PCD and asthma, personalized treatment strategies are essential. In PCD patients with a confirmed asthma diagnosis—characterized by elevated FeNO, atopy, or eosinophilia—a dual management approach may be necessary, incorporating both ICS and airway clearance therapies [126, 127]. Conversely, in patients without evidence of eosinophilic inflammation or with poor response to asthma medications, focus should remain on optimizing mucociliary clearance and infection control [121, 128].

Emerging endotyping strategies and biomarker profiling (e.g., nNO, FeNO, sputum cytology) may eventually guide therapy more precisely. The integration of pulmonary function trends, exacerbation history, and inflammatory patterns can support a phenotype-driven treatment plan, minimizing unnecessary medications and maximizing clinical outcomes.

Ultimately, therapeutic decision-making in PCD with overlapping asthma features should be individualized, based on objective testing, clinical response, and the predominant pathophysiological driver [14, 83, 86].

8. Current guidelines and limitations

While the clinical management of PCD and asthma is guided by international guidelines, significant limitations remain when these conditions overlap—whether as comorbidities or diagnostic mimics [14, 129]. This section reviews current recommendations and highlights the challenges clinicians face in dual diagnosis.

8.1 Review of ERS and ATS guidelines for PCD and asthma

The European Respiratory Society (ERS) and American Thoracic Society (ATS) have published comprehensive guidelines for the diagnosis and management of PCD [130]. These emphasize early diagnosis using a combination of nNO, high-speed video microscopy (HSVM), electron microscopy, immunofluorescence, and genetic testing. Once diagnosed, management centers on regular airway clearance therapy, monitoring for bronchiectasis progression, treatment of infections, and hearing surveillance. No specific anti-inflammatory agents are endorsed unless a clear coexisting diagnosis (such as asthma) is present.

In contrast, asthma guidelines from ERS, ATS, and GINA (Global Initiative for Asthma) focus on controlling airway inflammation with a stepwise approach to inhaled corticosteroids, bronchodilators, and biologic therapies based on severity and phenotype [73, 131, 132]. Asthma care emphasizes symptom control, prevention of exacerbations, and lung function preservation [133].

8.2 Lack of specific recommendations for dual-diagnosed patients

Despite overlapping features and increasing recognition of asthma diagnoses in PCD cohorts, current guidelines do not provide recommendations for managing patients with both conditions [130]. To date, there is no consensus on when to initiate corticosteroids or bronchodilators in PCD, nor on how to adjust airway clearance regimens in asthmatic patients with impaired mucociliary function [134, 135]. This gap creates clinical uncertainty, often leading to either overtreatment with asthma medications or undertreatment of airway obstruction in PCD.

8.3 Gaps in evidence and management algorithms

Few randomized controlled trials exist evaluating the effectiveness of asthma medications in PCD populations, and most treatment approaches are extrapolated from cystic fibrosis or non-PCD bronchiectasis guidelines [14, 83]. Moreover, phenotyping tools like FeNO or sputum eosinophil counts, commonly used in asthma management, are not well-validated in PCD [136, 137]. Similarly, biomarkers like nNO, although diagnostic in PCD, do not guide therapeutic decision-making [138].

There is also a paucity of longitudinal data on patients with coexisting asthma and PCD, making it difficult to assess the natural history, treatment response, or optimal timing for interventions [14]. This absence of tailored algorithms leads to fragmented care, particularly in children, where early differentiation between asthma and PCD is critical but challenging.

While guideline-based care exists for both PCD and asthma independently, there is a pressing need for research, clinical consensus, and integrated protocols that address the unique needs of patients who present with overlapping features or dual diagnoses. Until then, clinicians must rely on clinical judgment, multidisciplinary collaboration, and personalized treatment plans informed by objective testing and response to therapy.

9. Future directions in research and clinical practice

As the clinical and biological overlap between asthma and PCD becomes increasingly evident, the need to refine diagnostic tools and treatment paradigms has grown more urgent. Several avenues of research and innovation can help close current knowledge gaps and support more accurate, individualized patient care.

9.1 Need for longitudinal studies and registries

There is a pressing need for prospective, longitudinal studies that follow patients with PCD—both with and without asthma features—to better understand the natural history, disease progression, and response to therapy. While existing PCD registries, such as the international PCD (iPCD) cohort and the PCD Foundation Registry (PCDFR), have provided valuable cross-sectional insights, they are limited by heterogeneity in data collection and underrepresentation of comorbidities such as asthma [90]. Expanding these registries to include detailed phenotyping, lung function trajectories, medication use, and exacerbation frequency would allow for improved stratification of patients and identification of true overlap syndromes. Inclusion of early-life and neonatal data may also support efforts toward earlier diagnosis.

9.2 Biomarkers and imaging in distinguishing phenotypes

Distinguishing asthma from PCD—or identifying patients with both—requires reliable biomarkers and imaging techniques. Current asthma diagnostics utilize tools such as FeNO, serum IgE, and eosinophil counts [139], while PCD diagnosis relies heavily on nNO, ciliary ultrastructure, and genetics [140]. However, these modalities have limited sensitivity in overlap scenarios. Newer approaches, such as airway proteomics, inflammatory cytokine profiling, and advanced radiologic imaging (e.g., artificial intelligence-assisted CT analysis with 3D segmentation and reconstruction), hold promise in delineating phenotypic clusters and directing appropriate interventions [141–144]. Validation of these tools in diverse patient populations is a key research priority.

9.3 Integration of genomic data and precision medicine

Genetic sequencing is already a cornerstone of PCD diagnosis, with over 55 associated genes identified [145]. The integration of genomic data with clinical phenotypes, inflammatory markers, and treatment response could pave the way for a precision medicine approach to overlapping airway diseases [146]. Whole genome sequencing (WGS), transcriptomics, and epigenetic profiling may reveal shared molecular pathways or disease-modifying variants that contribute to airway hyperresponsiveness in PCD patients [145]. Similarly, machine learning applied to integrated omics data could facilitate the development of predictive models for treatment response or risk stratification [147]. Efforts to harmonize genetic databases and link them to clinical registries will be instrumental in realizing this goal. The future of care for patients with asthma and PCD lies in multidimensional research frameworks that unify clinical, molecular, and imaging data. Such efforts will enable more precise diagnoses, targeted treatments, and, ultimately, improved quality of life for patients navigating complex airway disease.

10. Conclusion

PCD and asthma are two distinct respiratory conditions with unique pathophysiological mechanisms, yet they often share overlapping clinical features, including chronic cough and airflow limitation. This overlap can lead to diagnostic uncertainty and treatment delays, especially in pediatric populations. Recent evidence suggests that a subset of PCD patients may exhibit asthma-like traits, including bronchodilator responsiveness and airway hyperreactivity, while many individuals with difficult-to-control "asthma" may in fact have underlying PCD that has not been identified.

This chapter has explored the key pathophysiological distinctions and intersections between PCD and asthma, with a focus on mucociliary dysfunction, inflammatory profiles, and biomarker expression. It also highlighted the current challenges in diagnosis, particularly in cases of nonresponsive asthma, and emphasized the importance of using objective tools—such as nNO, high-speed video microscopy, and genetic testing—to identify PCD early.

From a therapeutic standpoint, the cooccurrence of features from both diseases demands a personalized approach. While inhaled corticosteroids and bronchodilators may offer benefit in select patients with asthma features, the cornerstone of PCD management remains aggressive airway clearance and antimicrobial strategies. The integration of clinical phenotype, inflammatory endotype, and genetic information will be essential for guiding effective treatment.

Early recognition of PCD in patients with overlapping symptoms is critical to prevent irreversible lung damage. Multidisciplinary care involving pulmonologists, immunologists, otolaryngologists, and physiotherapists ensures a comprehensive approach to diagnosis and management. Moving forward, collaborative research, longitudinal registries, and biomarker-driven algorithms will be essential in improving outcomes for patients navigating this complex diagnostic and therapeutic interface.

Author details

Wilfredo De Jesús-Rojas[1]*, Gabriel Román-Ríos[1] and Ricardo A. Mosquera[2]

1 Department of Pediatrics and Basic Science, Ponce Health Science University, Ponce, PR, USA

2 Department of Pediatrics, McGovern Medical School, University of Texas Health Science Center at Houston, Houston, TX, USA

*Address all correspondence to: wdejesus@psm.edu

References

[1] Shapiro AJ, Davis SD, Polineni D, Manion M, Rosenfeld M, Dell SD, et al. Diagnosis of primary ciliary dyskinesia. An official American thoracic society clinical practice guideline. American Journal of Respiratory and Critical Care Medicine. 2018;**197**:e24-e39

[2] Knowles MR, Daniels LA, Davis SD, Zariwala MA, Leigh MW. Primary ciliary dyskinesia. Recent advances in diagnostics, genetics, and characterization of clinical disease. American Journal of Respiratory and Critical Care Medicine. 2013;**188**:913-922

[3] Zhao Y, Pinskey J, Lin J, Yin W, Sears PR, Daniels LA, et al. Structural insights into the cause of human RSPH4A primary ciliary dyskinesia. Molecular Biology of the Cell. 2021;**32**:1202-1209

[4] De Jesus-Rojas W, Shapiro AJ, Shoemark A. Respiratory aspects of primary ciliary dyskinesia. Clinics in Chest Medicine. 2024;**45**:717-728

[5] Marthin JK, Petersen N, Skovgaard LT, Nielsen KG. Lung function in patients with primary ciliary dyskinesia: A cross-sectional and 3-decade longitudinal study. American Journal of Respiratory and Critical Care Medicine. 2010;**181**:1262-1268

[6] Leigh MW, Pittman JE, Carson JL, Ferkol TW, Dell SD, Davis SD, et al. Clinical and genetic aspects of primary ciliary dyskinesia/Kartagener syndrome. Genetics in Medicine. 2009;**11**:473-487

[7] Yang C, Lv J, Li X, Yang X-T, Yin M-Y. Global burden of asthma in young adults in 204 countries and territories, 1990-2019: Systematic analysis of the global burden of disease study 2019. Preventive Medicine Reports. 2024;**37**:102531

[8] Habib N, Pasha MA, Tang DD. Current understanding of asthma pathogenesis and biomarkers. Cells. 2022;**11**:2764

[9] Hammad H, Lambrecht BN. The basic immunology of asthma. Cell. 2021;**184**:1469-1485

[10] Komlósi ZI, van de Veen W, Kovács N, Szűcs G, Sokolowska M, O'Mahony L, et al. Cellular and molecular mechanisms of allergic asthma. Molecular Aspects of Medicine. 2022;**85**:100995

[11] Boonpiyathad T, Sözener ZC, Satitsuksanoa P, Akdis CA. Immunologic mechanisms in asthma. Seminars in Immunology. 2019;**46**:101333

[12] Chen W, Puttock EJ, Xie F, Crawford W, Schatz M, Vollmer WM, et al. Symptoms of asthma extracted through natural language processing and their associations with acute asthma exacerbation in adults with mild asthma. The Journal of Allergy and Clinical Immunology. In Practice. 2025;S2213-2198(25)00389-7. [Advance Online Publication]. DOI: 10.1016/j.jaip.2025.04.031

[13] Yaghoubi M, Adibi A, Safari A, FitzGerald JM, Sadatsafavi M. The projected economic and health burden of uncontrolled asthma in the United States. American Journal of Respiratory and Critical Care Medicine. 2019;**200**:1102-1112

[14] Zein J, Owora A, Kim HJ, Marozkina N, Gaston B. Asthma among children with primary ciliary dyskinesia. JAMA Network Open. 2024;7:e2449795

[15] Olcese C, Patel MP, Shoemark A, Kiviluoto S, Legendre M, Williams HJ,

et al. X-linked primary ciliary dyskinesia due to mutations in the cytoplasmic axonemal dynein assembly factor PIH1D3. Nature Communications. 2017;**8**:14279

[16] Rezaei M, Soheili A, Ziai SA, Fakharian A, Toreyhi H, Pourabdollah M, et al. Transmission electron microscopy study of suspected primary ciliary dyskinesia patients. Scientific Reports. 2022;**12**:2375

[17] Davis SD, Rosenfeld M, Lee H-S, Ferkol TW, Sagel SD, Dell SD, et al. Primary ciliary dyskinesia: Longitudinal study of lung disease by ultrastructure defect and genotype. American Journal of Respiratory and Critical Care Medicine. 2019;**199**:190-198

[18] Smith EF, Yang P. The radial spokes and central apparatus: Mechano-chemical transducers that regulate flagellar motility. Cell Motility and the Cytoskeleton. 2004;**57**:8-17

[19] Grossman-Haham I, Coudray N, Yu Z, Wang F, Zhang N, Bhabha G, et al. Structure of the radial spoke head and insights into its role in mechanoregulation of ciliary beating. Nature Structural & Molecular Biology. 2021;**28**:20-28

[20] Arora S, Rana M, Sachdev A, D'Souza JS. Appearing and disappearing acts of cilia. Journal of Biosciences. 2023;**48**:8

[21] Theegarten D, Ebsen M. Ultrastructural pathology of primary ciliary dyskinesia: Report about 125 cases in Germany. Diagnostic Pathology. 2011;**6**:115

[22] Shapiro AJ, Leigh MW. Value of transmission electron microscopy for primary ciliary dyskinesia diagnosis in the era of molecular medicine: Genetic defects with normal and non-diagnostic ciliary ultrastructure. Ultrastructural Pathology. 2017;**41**:373-385

[23] Leigh MW, Horani A, Kinghorn B, O'Connor MG, Zariwala MA, Knowles MR. Primary ciliary dyskinesia (PCD): A genetic disorder of motile cilia. Translational Science of Rare Diseases. 2019;**4**:51-75

[24] Lobo J, Zariwala MA, Noone PG. Primary ciliary dyskinesia. Seminars in Respiratory and Critical Care Medicine. 2015;**36**:169-179

[25] De Jesús-Rojas W, Meléndez-Montañez J, Muñiz-Hernández J, Marra-Nazario A, Alvarado-Huerta F, Santos-López A, et al. The RSPH4A gene in primary ciliary dyskinesia. International Journal of Molecular Sciences. 2023;**24**:1936

[26] De Jesús-Rojas W, Muñiz-Hernández J, Alvarado-Huerta F, Meléndez-Montañez JM, Santos-López AJ, Mosquera RA. The genetics of primary ciliary dyskinesia in Puerto Rico. Diagnostics (Basel). 2022;**12**:1127

[27] Raidt J, Riepenhausen S, Pennekamp P, Olbrich H, Amirav I, Athanazio RA, et al. Analyses of 1236 genotyped primary ciliary dyskinesia individuals identify regional clusters of distinct DNA variants and significant genotype–phenotype correlations. The European Respiratory Journal. 2024;**64**:2301769

[28] De Jesús-Rojas W, Demetriou ZJ, Muñiz-Hernández J, Rosario-Ortiz G, Quiñones FM, Ramos-Benitez MJ, et al. Advancing primary ciliary dyskinesia diagnosis through high-speed video microscopy analysis. Cells. 2024;**13**:567

[29] Gileles-Hillel A, Mor-Shaked H, Shoseyov D, Reiter J, Tsabari R, Hevroni A, et al. Whole-exome

sequencing accuracy in the diagnosis of primary ciliary dyskinesia. ERJ Open Research. 2020;**6**(4):00213-2020. DOI: 10.1183/23120541.00213-2020

[30] Chilvers MA, Rutman A, O'Callaghan C. Ciliary beat pattern is associated with specific ultrastructural defects in primary ciliary dyskinesia. The Journal of Allergy and Clinical Immunology. 2003;**112**:518-524

[31] Pereira R, Barbosa T, Cardoso AL, Sá R, Sousa M. Cystic fibrosis and primary ciliary dyskinesia: Similarities and differences. Respiratory Medicine. 2023;**209**:107169

[32] McShane PJ, Naureckas ET, Tino G, Strek ME. Non-cystic fibrosis bronchiectasis. American Journal of Respiratory and Critical Care Medicine. 2013;**188**:647-656

[33] Shen C, Shen Y, Huang W, Zhang A, Zou T, Guo D, et al. A novel homozygous RSPH4A variant in a family with primary ciliary dyskinesia and literature review. Frontiers in Genetics. 2024;**15**:1364476

[34] Shoemark A, Frost E, Dixon M, Ollosson S, Kilpin K, Patel M, et al. Accuracy of immunofluorescence in the diagnosis of primary ciliary dyskinesia. American Journal of Respiratory and Critical Care Medicine. 2017;**196**:94-101

[35] Moldoveanu B, Otmishi P, Jani P, Walker J, Sarmiento X, Guardiola J, et al. Inflammatory mechanisms in the lung. Journal of Inflammation Research. 2009;**2**:1-11

[36] King PT. The pathophysiology of bronchiectasis. International Journal of Chronic Obstructive Pulmonary Disease. 2009;**4**:411-419

[37] Sagel SD, Davis SD, Campisi P, Dell SD. Update of respiratory tract disease in children with primary ciliary dyskinesia. Proceedings of the American Thoracic Society. 2011;**8**:438-443

[38] Collison R, Hyatali SA, Kamenova A, Rashed A, Riley D, Kumar K, et al. Primary ciliary dyskinesia: Aetiology, diagnosis and clinical management. Clinical Medicine. 2025;**25**:100319

[39] Mullowney T, Manson D, Kim R, Stephens D, Shah V, Dell S. Primary ciliary dyskinesia and neonatal respiratory distress. Pediatrics. 2014;**134**:1160-1166

[40] Popatia R, Haver K, Casey A. Primary ciliary dyskinesia: An update on new diagnostic modalities and review of the literature. Pediatric Allergy, Immunology and Pulmonology. 2014;**27**:51-59

[41] O'Connor MG, Mosquera R, Metjian H, Marmor M, Olivier KN, Shapiro AJ. Primary ciliary dyskinesia. CHEST Pulmonary. 2023;**1**(1):100004. DOI: 10.1016/j.chpulm.2023.100004

[42] Pruliere-Escabasse V, Coste A, Chauvin P, Fauroux B, Tamalet A, Garabedian EN, et al. Otologic features in children with primary ciliary dyskinesia. Archives of Otolaryngology – Head & Neck Surgery. 2010;**136**:1121-1126

[43] Günaydın RÖ, Eroğlu E, Tellioğlu B, Emiralioğlu N, Özçelik HU, Yalçın E, et al. Evaluation of otorhinolaryngological manifestations in patients with primary ciliary dyskinesia. International Journal of Pediatric Otorhinolaryngology. 2023;**168**:111520

[44] Mirra V, Werner C, Santamaria F. Primary ciliary dyskinesia: An update on clinical aspects, genetics, diagnosis, and future treatment strategies. Frontiers in Pediatrics. 2017;**5**:135

[45] Bradley J, Moran F, Greenstone M. Physical training for bronchiectasis. Cochrane Database of Systematic Reviews. 2002;**2002**:CD002166

[46] Svobodová T, Djakow J, Zemková D, Cipra A, Pohunek P, Lebl J. Impaired growth during childhood in patients with primary ciliary dyskinesia. International Journal of Endocrinology. 2013;**2013**:731423

[47] Sarkar M, Mahesh DM, Madabhavi I. Digital clubbing. Lung India. 2012;**29**:354-362

[48] Balbino M, Montatore M, Masino F, Guglielmi G. Kartagener's syndrome: A rare condition diagnosed in a young male patient. Radiology Case Reports. 2024;**19**:2741-2744

[49] Barber AT, Shapiro AJ, Davis SD, Ferkol TW, Atkinson JJ, Sagel SD, et al. Laterality defects in primary ciliary dyskinesia: Relationship to ultrastructural defect or genotype. Annals of the American Thoracic Society. 2023;**20**:397-405

[50] Shapiro AJ, Davis SD, Ferkol T, Dell SD, Rosenfeld M, Olivier KN, et al. Laterality defects other than situs inversus totalis in primary ciliary dyskinesia: Insights into situs ambiguus and heterotaxy. Chest. 2014;**146**:1176-1186

[51] Forrest K, Barricella AC, Pohar SA, Hinman AM, Amack JD. Understanding laterality disorders and the left-right organizer: Insights from zebrafish. Frontiers in Cell and Development Biology. 2022;**10**:1035513

[52] Whitfield M, Thomas L, Bequignon E, Schmitt A, Stouvenel L, Montantin G, et al. Mutations in DNAH17, encoding a sperm-specific axonemal outer dynein arm heavy chain, cause isolated male infertility due to Asthenozoospermia. American Journal of Human Genetics. 2019;**105**:198-212

[53] Gaude GS. Pulmonary manifestations of gastroesophageal reflux disease. Annals of Thoracic Medicine. 2009;**4**:115-123

[54] Lee AL, Goldstein RS. Gastroesophageal reflux disease in COPD: Links and risks. International Journal of Chronic Obstructive Pulmonary Disease. 2015;**10**:1935-1949

[55] Bradding P, Porsbjerg C, Côté A, Dahlén S-E, Hallstrand TS, Brightling CE. Airway hyperresponsiveness in asthma: The role of the epithelium. Journal of Allergy and Clinical Immunology. 2024;**153**:1181-1193

[56] Goldin J, Hashmi MF, Cataletto ME. Asthma. In: StatPearls. Treasure Island. FL: StatPearls Publishing; 2025

[57] Kuruvilla ME, Lee FE-H, Lee GB. Understanding asthma phenotypes, endotypes, and mechanisms of disease. Clinical Reviews in Allergy and Immunology. 2019;**56**:219-233

[58] Yue M, Gaietto K, Han YY, Rosser FJ, Xu Z, Qoyawayma C, et al. Transcriptomic profiles in nasal epithelium and asthma endotypes in youth. JAMA. 2025;**333**:307

[59] Taunk ST, Cardet JC, Ledford DK. Clinical implications of asthma endotypes and phenotypes. Allergy and Asthma Proceedings. 2022;**43**:375-382

[60] Lloyd CM, Hessel EM. Functions of T cells in asthma: More than just T(H)2 cells. Nature Reviews. Immunology. 2010;**10**:838-848

[61] León B. Understanding the development of Th2 cell-driven allergic

airway disease in early life. Frontiers in Allergy. 2022;**3**:1080153

[62] Bosnjak B, Stelzmueller B, Erb KJ, Epstein MM. Treatment of allergic asthma: Modulation of Th2 cells and their responses. Respiratory Research. 2011;**12**:114

[63] Indolfi C, Klain A, Capuano MC, Colosimo S, Rapillo R, Miraglia Del Giudice M. Severe asthma in school-age children: An updated appraisal on biological options and challenges in this age group. Children. 2025;**12**:167

[64] Hudey SN, Ledford DK, Cardet JC. Mechanisms of non-type 2 asthma. Current Opinion in Immunology. 2020;**66**:123-128

[65] Sze E, Bhalla A, Nair P. Mechanisms and therapeutic strategies for non-T2 asthma. Allergy. 2020;**75**:311-325

[66] Xie Y, Abel PW, Casale TB, Tu Y. TH17 cells and corticosteroid insensitivity in severe asthma. The Journal of Allergy and Clinical Immunology. 2022;**149**:467-479

[67] Hinks TSC, Levine SJ, Brusselle GG. Treatment options in type-2 low asthma. The European Respiratory Journal. 2021;**57**:2000528

[68] Gillissen A, Paparoupa M. Inflammation and infections in asthma. The Clinical Respiratory Journal. 2015;**9**:257-269

[69] Varricchi G, Brightling CE, Grainge C, Lambrecht BN, Chanez P. Airway remodelling in asthma and the epithelium: On the edge of a new era. The European Respiratory Journal. 2024;**63**:2301619

[70] Pelaia G, Vatrella A, Busceti MT, Gallelli L, Calabrese C, Terracciano R, et al. Cellular mechanisms underlying eosinophilic and neutrophilic airway inflammation in asthma. Mediators of Inflammation. 2015;**2015**:879783

[71] Kistemaker LEM, Oenema TA, Meurs H, Gosens R. Regulation of airway inflammation and remodeling by muscarinic receptors: Perspectives on anticholinergic therapy in asthma and COPD. Life Sciences. 2012;**91**:1126-1133

[72] Hough KP, Curtiss ML, Blain TJ, Liu R-M, Trevor J, Deshane JS, et al. Airway remodeling in asthma. Frontiers in Medicine (Lausanne). 2020;**7**:191

[73] Global Initiative for Asthma. Global Strategy for Asthma Management and Prevention; 2024. Available from: https://ginasthma.org/2024-report/

[74] Miculinić A, Mrkić Kobal I, Kušan T, Turkalj M, Plavec D. Current challenges in pediatric asthma. Children (Basel). 2024;**11**:632

[75] Kim SR, Rhee YK. Overlap between asthma and COPD: Where the two diseases converge. Allergy, Asthma & Immunology Research. 2010;**2**:209-214

[76] Kavanagh J, Jackson DJ, Kent BD. Over- and under-diagnosis in asthma. Breathe (Sheffield, England). 2019;**15**:e20-e27

[77] Aaron SD, Vandemheen KL, FitzGerald JM, Ainslie M, Gupta S, Lemière C, et al. Reevaluation of diagnosis in adults with physician-diagnosed asthma. JAMA. 2017;**317**:269

[78] de Benedictis FM. GPs meet rare lung disorders task force factsheet: Primary ciliary dyskinesia. Breathe (Sheffield, England). 2015;**11**:159-161

[79] Papi A, Brightling C, Pedersen SE, Reddel HK. Asthma. Lancet. 2018;**391**: 783-800

[80] Doeing DC, Solway J. Airway smooth muscle in the pathophysiology and treatment of asthma. Journal of Applied Physiology. 1985;**2013**(114):834-843

[81] Frohlich M, Prentice B, Owens L, Waters S, Morgan L. Beyond the present: Current and future perspectives on the role of infections in pediatric PCD. Frontiers in Pediatrics. 2025;**13**:1564156

[82] Polverino E, Dimakou K, Hurst J, Martinez-Garcia M-A, Miravitlles M, Paggiaro P, et al. The overlap between bronchiectasis and chronic airway diseases: State of the art and future directions. The European Respiratory Journal. 2018;**52**:1800328

[83] Marozkina N. Ciliary function, antigen stasis and asthma. IJMS. 2024;**25**:10043

[84] Hosoki K, Fujisawa T, Masuda S, Usui S, Ito H, Nagao M, et al. A case of primary ciliary dyskinesia who had been treated as asthma. Arerugī. 2010;**59**:847-854

[85] Barbato A, Frischer T, Kuehni CE, Snijders D, Azevedo I, Baktai G, et al. Primary ciliary dyskinesia: A consensus statement on diagnostic and treatment approaches in children. The European Respiratory Journal. 2009;**34**:1264-1276

[86] Lucas JS, Barbato A, Collins SA, Goutaki M, Behan L, Caudri D, et al. European respiratory society guidelines for the diagnosis of primary ciliary dyskinesia. The European Respiratory Journal. 2017;**49**(1):1601090. DOI: 10.1183/13993003.01090-2016

[87] De Jesus-Rojas W, Alvarado-Huerta F, Melendez-Montanez JM, Muniz-Hernandez J, Santos-Lopez A, Mosquera RA. Nasal nitric oxide levels: Improving the diagnosis of primary ciliary dyskinesia in Puerto Rico. Advances in Respiratory Medicine. 2022;**90**:399-406

[88] Werner C, Onnebrink JG, Omran H. Diagnosis and management of primary ciliary dyskinesia. Cilia. 2015;**4**:2

[89] Levine H, Bar-On O, Nir V, West N, Dizitzer Y, Mussaffi H, et al. Reversible bronchial obstruction in primary ciliary dyskinesia. Journal of Clinical Medicine. 2022;**11**:6791

[90] Goutaki M, Maurer E, Halbeisen FS, Amirav I, Barbato A, Behan L, et al. The international primary ciliary dyskinesia cohort (iPCD cohort): Methods and first results. The European Respiratory Journal. 2017;**49**:1601181

[91] Leal-Jiménez E, Avilés-Ramírez BA, Reyes-Rosales M. Discinesia ciliar primaria. Causa de infecciones respiratorias recurrentes: serie de tres casos. NCT Neumología y Cirugía de Tórax. 2023;**82**:38-41

[92] Takeuchi K, Xu Y, Ogawa S, Ikejiri M, Nakatani K, Gotoh S, et al. A pediatric case of productive cough caused by novel variants in DNAH9. Human Genome Variation. 2021;**8**:3

[93] Tong L, Li L, Wang W, Chen J. Case report: Primary ciliary dyskinesia due to CCNO mutations: A Chinese pediatric case series and literature review. Frontiers in Pediatrics. 2024;**12**:1458660

[94] Leigh MW, Zariwala MA, Knowles MR. Primary ciliary dyskinesia: Improving the diagnostic approach. Current Opinion in Pediatrics. 2009;**21**:320-325

[95] Gravesande KSV, Omran H. Primary ciliary dyskinesia: Clinical presentation, diagnosis and genetics. Annals of Medicine. 2005;**37**:439-449

[96] George L, Brightling CE. Eosinophilic airway inflammation: Role in asthma and chronic obstructive pulmonary disease. Therapeutic Advances in Chronic Disease. 2016;7:34-51

[97] Sagel SD, Kupfer O, Wagner BD, Davis SD, Dell SD, Ferkol TW, et al. Airway inflammation in children with primary ciliary dyskinesia. Annals of the American Thoracic Society. 2023;**20**:67-74

[98] Eralp EE, Karadag B. Recent advances in primary ciliary dyskinesia: From diagnosis to treatment. US Respiratory & Pulmonary Diseases. 2021;**6**:14

[99] Rimmer J. Congenital problems of mucociliary clearance: Primary ciliary dyskinesia. Rhinology. 2012;**50**:353-359

[100] Horton K, Wing PAC, Jackson CL, McCormick CJ, Carroll MP, Lucas JS. Interplay between respiratory viruses and cilia in the airways. European Respiratory Review. 2025;**34**:240224

[101] Mehta K. Primary ciliary dyskinesia: A review. Canadian Allergy & Immunology Today. 2021;**1**(3):34-40. DOI: 10.58931/cait.2021.1323

[102] Livraghi-Butrico A, Kelly EJ, Klem ER, Dang H, Wolfgang MC, Boucher RC, et al. Mucus clearance, MyD88-dependent and MyD88-independent immunity modulate lung susceptibility to spontaneous bacterial infection and inflammation. Mucosal Immunology. 2012;**5**:397-408

[103] Raby KL, Michaeloudes C, Tonkin J, Chung KF, Bhavsar PK. Mechanisms of airway epithelial injury and abnormal repair in asthma and COPD. Frontiers in Immunology. 2023;**14**:1201658

[104] Russell RJ, Boulet L-P, Brightling CE, Pavord ID, Porsbjerg C, Dorscheid D, et al. The airway epithelium: An orchestrator of inflammation, a key structural barrier and a therapeutic target in severe asthma. The European Respiratory Journal. 2024;**63**:2301397

[105] Gatt D, Ratjen F. Preventing continuous damage in primary ciliary dyskinesia: Is airway inflammation a potential target? Annals of the American Thoracic Society. 2023;**20**:26-27

[106] Chalmers JD, Metersky M, Aliberti S, Morgan L, Fucile S, Lauterio M, et al. Neutrophilic inflammation in bronchiectasis. European Respiratory Review. 2025;**34**:240179

[107] Voynow JA, Shinbashi M. Neutrophil elastase and chronic lung disease. Biomolecules. 2021;**11**:1065

[108] Lambrecht BN, Hammad H, Fahy JV. The cytokines of asthma. Immunity. 2019;**50**:975-991

[109] Ilmarinen P, Tuomisto LE, Kankaanranta H. Phenotypes, risk factors, and mechanisms of adult-onset asthma. Mediators of Inflammation. 2015;**2015**:514868

[110] Paternò S, Pisani L, Zanconato S, Ferraro VA, Carraro S. Role of nasal nitric oxide in primary ciliary dyskinesia and other respiratory conditions in children. International Journal of Molecular Sciences. 2023;**24**:16159

[111] Louca N, Damianou D, Kostea N, Kouis P, Yiallouros P, Pitsios C. Assessing nasal nitric oxide in allergic rhinitis: A controversial biomarker. Medicina (Kaunas, Lithuania). 2025;**61**:516

[112] Shapiro AJ, Dell SD, Gaston B, O'Connor M, Marozkina N, Manion M, et al. Nasal nitric oxide measurement in primary ciliary dyskinesia. A technical paper on standardized testing protocols.

Annals of the American Thoracic Society. 2020;**17**:e1-e12

[113] Maniscalco M, Fuschillo S, Mormile I, Detoraki A, Sarnelli G, Paulis A, et al. Exhaled nitric oxide as biomarker of type 2 diseases. Cells. 2023;**12**:2518

[114] Pignatti P, Visca D, Loukides S, Märtson A-G, Alffenaar J-WC, Migliori GB, et al. A snapshot of exhaled nitric oxide and asthma characteristics: Experience from high to low income countries. Pulmonology. 2022;**28**:44-58

[115] Nielsen KG, Holgersen MG, Crowley S, Marthin JK. Chronic airway disease in primary ciliary dyskinesia—Spiced with geno–phenotype associations. American Journal of Medical Genetics Part C. 2022;**190**:20-35

[116] Werner C, Onnebrink JG, Omran H. Diagnosis and management of primary ciliary dyskinesia. Cilia. 2015;**4**(1):2. DOI: 10.1186/s13630-014-0011-8

[117] Phillips G, Thomas S, Heather S, Bush A. Airway response of children with primary ciliary dyskinesia to exercise and beta2-agonist challenge. The European Respiratory Journal. 1998;**11**:1389-1391

[118] Fauroux B, Tamalet A, Clément A. Management of primary ciliary dyskinesia: The lower airways. Paediatric Respiratory Reviews. 2009;**10**:55-57

[119] Paff T, Omran H, Nielsen KG, Haarman EG. Current and future treatments in primary ciliary dyskinesia. International Journal of Molecular Sciences. 2021;**22**(18):9834. DOI: 10.3390/ijms22189834

[120] Bennett WD, Henderson AG, Ceppe A, Zeman KL, Wu J, Gladman C, et al. Effect of hypertonic saline on mucociliary clearance and clinical outcomes in chronic bronchitis. ERJ Open Research. 2020;**6**:00269-02020

[121] Schofield LM, Duff A, Brennan C. Airway clearance techniques for primary ciliary dyskinesia; is the cystic fibrosis literature portable? Paediatric Respiratory Reviews. 2018;**25**:73-77

[122] Qiu S, Zhong X. Macrolides: A promising pharmacologic therapy for chronic obstructive pulmonary disease. Therapeutic Advances in Respiratory Disease. 2017;**11**:147-155

[123] Kobbernagel HE, Buchvald FF, Haarman EG, Casaulta C, Collins SA, Hogg C, et al. Efficacy and safety of azithromycin maintenance therapy in primary ciliary dyskinesia (BESTCILIA): A multicentre, double-blind, randomised, placebo-controlled phase 3 trial. The Lancet Respiratory Medicine. 2020;**8**:493-505

[124] Steel HC, Theron AJ, Cockeran R, Anderson R, Feldman C. Pathogen- and host-directed anti-inflammatory activities of macrolide antibiotics. Mediators of Inflammation. 2012;**2012**:1-17

[125] Crosbie PAJ, Woodhead MA. Long-term macrolide therapy in chronic inflammatory airway diseases. The European Respiratory Journal. 2009;**33**:171-181

[126] Gremmo ML, Guenza MC. Positive expiratory pressure in the physiotherapeutic management of primary ciliary dyskinesia in paediatric age. Monaldi Archives for Chest Disease. 1999;**54**:255-257

[127] Barnes PJ. Inhaled corticosteroids. Pharmaceuticals (Basel). 2010;**3**:514-540

[128] Shapiro AJ, Zariwala MA, Ferkol T, Davis SD, Sagel SD, Dell SD, et al.

Diagnosis, monitoring, and treatment of primary ciliary dyskinesia: PCD foundation consensus recommendations based on state of the art review. Pediatric Pulmonology. 2016;**51**:115-132

[129] Ullmann N, Mirra V, Di Marco A, Pavone M, Porcaro F, Negro V, et al. Asthma: Differential diagnosis and comorbidities. Frontiers in Pediatrics. 2018;**6**:276

[130] Shoemark A, Dell S, Shapiro A, Lucas JS. ERS and ATS diagnostic guidelines for primary ciliary dyskinesia: Similarities and differences in approach to diagnosis. The European Respiratory Journal. 2019;**54**:1901066

[131] Louis R, Satia I, Ojanguren I, Schleich F, Bonini M, Tonia T, et al. European Respiratory Society guidelines for the diagnosis of asthma in adults. The European Respiratory Journal. 2022;**60**:2101585

[132] Reddel HK, Bacharier LB, Bateman ED, Brightling CE, Brusselle GG, Buhl R, et al. Global initiative for asthma strategy 2021: Executive summary and rationale for key changes. American Journal of Respiratory and Critical Care Medicine. 2022;**205**:17-35

[133] Castillo JR, Peters SP, Busse WW. Asthma exacerbations: Pathogenesis, prevention, and treatment. The Journal of Allergy and Clinical Immunology. In Practice. 2017;**5**:918-927

[134] Dehlink E, Richardson C, Marsh G, Lee K, Jamalzadeh A, Bush A, et al. Are inhaled corticosteroids prescribed rationally in primary ciliary dyskinesia? The European Respiratory Journal. 2018;**51**:1702221

[135] Jesenak M, Durdik P, Oppova D, Franova S, Diamant Z, Golebski K, et al. Dysfunctional mucociliary clearance in asthma and airway remodeling—New insights into an old topic. Respiratory Medicine. 2023;**218**:107372

[136] Wagener AH, De Nijs SB, Lutter R, Sousa AR, Weersink EJM, Bel EH, et al. External validation of blood eosinophils, FENO and serum periostin as surrogates for sputum eosinophils in asthma. Thorax. 2015;**70**:115-120

[137] Dweik RA, Boggs PB, Erzurum SC, Irvin CG, Leigh MW, Lundberg JO, et al. An official ATS clinical practice guideline: Interpretation of exhaled nitric oxide levels (FENO) for clinical applications. American Journal of Respiratory and Critical Care Medicine. 2011;**184**:602-615

[138] Saunders JL, O'Connor MG, Machogu EM. Nasal nitric oxide May not differentiate primary ciliary dyskinesia from certain primary immunodeficiencies. Pediatric Pulmonology. 2022;**57**(9):2269-2272. DOI: 10.1002/ppul.25989

[139] Badar A, Salem AM, Bamosa AO, Qutub HO, Gupta RK, Siddiqui IA. Association between FeNO, Total blood IgE, peripheral blood eosinophil and inflammatory cytokines in partly controlled asthma. Journal of Asthma and Allergy. 2020;**13**:533-543

[140] Leigh MW, O'Callaghan C, Knowles MR. The challenges of diagnosing primary ciliary dyskinesia. Proceedings of the American Thoracic Society. 2011;**8**:434-437

[141] Wu Y, Xia S, Liang Z, Chen R, Qi S. Artificial intelligence in COPD CT images: Identification, staging, and quantitation. Respiratory Research. 2024;**25**:319

[142] Polley DJ, Latham P, Choi MY, Buhler KA, Fritzler MJ, Fritzler ML.

Identification of novel clusters of co-expressing cytokines in a diagnostic cytokine multiplex test. Frontiers in Immunology. 2023;**14**:1223817

[143] Schofield JPR, Burg D, Nicholas B, Strazzeri F, Brandsma J, Staykova D, et al. Stratification of asthma phenotypes by airway proteomic signatures. The Journal of Allergy and Clinical Immunology. 2019;**144**:70-82

[144] Agache I, Shamji MH, Kermani NZ, Vecchi G, Favaro A, Layhadi JA, et al. Multidimensional endotyping using nasal proteomics predicts molecular phenotypes in the asthmatic airways. Journal of Allergy and Clinical Immunology. 2023;**151**:128-137

[145] Black HA, de Proce SM, Campos JL, Meynert A, Halachev M, Marsh JA, et al. Whole genome sequencing enhances molecular diagnosis of primary ciliary dyskinesia. Pediatric Pulmonology. 2024;**59**:3322-3332

[146] Mani S, Lalani SR, Pammi M. Genomics and multiomics in the age of precision medicine. Pediatric Research. 2025;**97**:1399-1410

[147] Sharma A, Lysenko A, Jia S, Boroevich KA, Tsunoda T. Advances in AI and machine learning for predictive medicine. Journal of Human Genetics. 2024;**69**:487-497

Section 4

Difficulties to Manage Asthma

Chapter 5

Severe Asthma: Phenotypes, Endotypes and Therapeutic Response

Stefan-Marian Frent

Abstract

Severe asthma, defined as asthma that remains uncontrolled despite receiving optimized treatment with high-dose inhaled corticosteroids and long-acting bronchodilators (ICS/LABA), or that requires such treatment to avoid becoming uncontrolled, is linked to a heightened risk of severe exacerbations and death, and accounts for a significant portion of the total costs associated with asthma care. Asthma phenotypes and endotypes are two essential concepts that help enhance our understanding of the diversity within the asthma population. Phenotyping involves classifying individuals based on observable clinical and biological traits. In contrast, endotyping provides a deeper understanding of the molecular and biological mechanisms driving asthma by identifying specific pathways and biomarkers associated with the disease. By targeting specific molecular mechanisms underlying airway inflammation in severe asthma, biologic therapy has emerged as a disease-modifying treatment, allowing for the development of the concept of asthma remission.

Keywords: severe asthma, T2-inflammation, biologics, phenotype, endotype

1. Introduction

Asthma is a common airway disease, with an estimated prevalence ranging from 1 to 29% of the population in different countries. Typical symptoms include persistent cough, wheezing, recurrent dyspnea, and chest tightness, with variations in intensity and over time, usually accompanied by variable airflow limitation [1].

Asthma is considered a heterogeneous syndrome, with multiple phenotypes described, such as allergic asthma, adult-onset asthma, occupational asthma, cough-variant asthma, and asthma in obese patients. These phenotypes emerge at the interplay between environmental triggers (allergens, viral infections, pollutants, etc.) and the host immune response, strongly influenced by genetic characteristics. Airway inflammation and hyperresponsiveness are considered the two key hallmarks of asthma.

The respiratory epithelium is increasingly recognized as playing a central role in the priming and persistence of an abnormal inflammatory T2 response to the above-mentioned environmental stimuli. Airway inflammation involves numerous cell types, mediators, and downstream immune pathways [2–4], and is responsible for increased asthma symptoms [2, 3]. Multiple inflammatory endotypes have been identified [4]. Airway hyperresponsiveness is an intricate interplay of airway inflammation, airway remodeling, and airway smooth muscle hypercontractility [5]. The severity of airway hyperresponsiveness has also been associated with increased asthma symptoms [6].

2. Severe asthma

Severe asthma represents a distinct clinical subset within the broader asthma population, accounting for approximately 3–5% of all patients yet contributing disproportionately to healthcare utilization, morbidity, and mortality. According to the European Respiratory Society (ERS) and American Thoracic Society (ATS) guidelines, severe asthma is defined as asthma that requires treatment with high-dose inhaled corticosteroids (ICS) plus a second controller (and/or systemic corticosteroids) to prevent it from becoming uncontrolled or that remains uncontrolled despite this therapy [7]. This definition assumes adequate adherence, optimized inhaler technique, and appropriate management of comorbidities [1].

Uncontrolled asthma is characterized by frequent symptoms, persistent airflow limitation, two or more exacerbations requiring oral corticosteroids per year, or one or more asthma-related hospitalizations. Severe asthma should be differentiated from difficult-to-treat asthma, which may become controllable once modifiable factors, such as poor adherence, environmental triggers, or incorrect diagnosis, are addressed.

Heterogeneity in clinical presentation and pathophysiology has prompted a shift from a one-size-fits-all approach to a focus on phenotyping and endotyping, allowing for more personalized, biomarker-driven management strategies [8].

The classification of severe asthma into phenotypes and endotypes has enabled the development of personalized management strategies. The most widely recognized distinction is between type 2 (T2)-high and T2-low inflammation. T2-high asthma, marked by elevated eosinophils, FeNO, and IgE, often responds to corticosteroids and targeted biologics [9]. T2-low asthma, on the other hand, involves neutrophilic or paucigranulocytic inflammation, tends to be steroid-resistant, and lacks clear biomarkers or effective targeted therapies [10].

Airway remodeling, persistent inflammation, and immune dysregulation are key components of the pathophysiology of severe asthma. In T2-high asthma, cytokines such as IL-4, IL-5, and IL-13 drive eosinophilic inflammation. In T2-low asthma, IL-17 and TNF-alpha are more prominent, with an innate immune response resistant to corticosteroid treatment [11]. Remodeling includes thickened basement membrane, smooth muscle hypertrophy, and mucous metaplasia, often independent of inflammatory cell counts [8].

The concept of treatable traits emphasizes the identification of specific clinical, inflammatory, and physiological traits—such as eosinophilia, chronic rhinosinusitis, and obesity—that can guide targeted therapy. Biologics, such as omalizumab (anti-IgE), mepolizumab and benralizumab (anti-IL-5), and dupilumab (anti-IL-4Rα), have significantly reduced exacerbation rates in patients with T2-high severe asthma [12, 13]. Tezepelumab, an anti-TSLP biologic, offers promise for broader applicability across endotypes [14].

3. Asthma phenotypes

3.1 The shift toward phenotypic classification

Traditionally, asthma was diagnosed and managed based on symptom patterns and lung function tests. However, growing evidence has shown that patients with similar symptoms can have vastly different inflammatory profiles, responses to therapy, and clinical outcomes. This has led to an explosion of data-driven phenotyping studies aimed at delineating meaningful subgroups.

A systematic review of 68 clustering studies in adult populations revealed significant heterogeneity in asthma phenotypes [15]. The most commonly identified patterns were associated with atopy, gender, and disease severity. These data-driven approaches highlight how asthma cannot be reduced to a single disease entity, but rather represents a spectrum of disorders driven by distinct biological mechanisms.

3.2 Clinical and molecular phenotypes

Several phenotypes have been consistently reported in the literature. One comprehensive review categorized adult asthma into four broad clinical subtypes: (1) early-onset mild allergic asthma, (2) moderate-to-severe allergic remodeling asthma, (3) late-onset allergic non-eosinophilic asthma, and (4) late-onset allergic eosinophilic asthma. Another clustering analysis supported five robust phenotypes, ranging from mild early-onset allergic forms to severe, late-onset, non-allergic asthma with fixed airway obstruction.

Importantly, these phenotypes correspond with specific molecular endotypes, particularly the distinction between type 2 (T2)-high and T2-low asthma. This classification is central to both pathophysiological understanding and therapeutic decision-making.

A disease phenotype refers to the set of clinically observable features of a condition, without necessarily reflecting the underlying biological mechanisms. In contrast, endotypes represent subtypes of a disease that are defined by distinct pathophysiological processes. In the context of asthma, phenotypes encompass clinical presentation, morphological traits, and variations in treatment response. While phenotypes are useful for guiding clinical decisions based on symptom patterns and triggers, they do not inherently provide insight into the disease's molecular basis [16].

Asthma endotypes, on the other hand, are characterized by specific cellular and molecular mechanisms, including interactions between immune pathways and airway structural cells. Identifying these mechanisms offers a deeper understanding of the disease and enables classification through the use of biomarkers derived from body fluids or affected tissues [17]. This mechanism-based classification, or endotyping, holds promise for advancing personalized asthma management, potentially improving therapeutic outcomes by targeting the specific biological drivers of the disease [18, 19].

Early efforts to classify asthma phenotypes focused primarily on patients' clinical and functional characteristics, without accounting for the underlying molecular profiles. However, it is now recognized that each phenotype is driven by a complex interplay of multiple molecular pathways, often referred to as the "molecular phenotype" [20]. When a specific and well-defined biological pathway is found to fully explain the clinical features of a given phenotype, this subset is designated an endotype—a concept first introduced by Anderson [18].

The origins of asthma phenotyping trace back to the late 1940s, when Rackemann [21] proposed two distinct forms of asthma: "extrinsic," primarily associated with atopy, and "intrinsic," which lacked any apparent allergic component. However, later studies highlighted more similarities than differences between these categories [22, 23], ultimately leading to the decline of the extrinsic/intrinsic classification in modern practice.

Robinson et al. identified two subsets of T-lymphocytes—T-helper (Th) 1 and Th2 cells—based on distinct cytokine mRNA expression profiles [24]. Notably, Th2 cells were found to be predominantly active in patients with atopic asthma. This discovery marked a pivotal moment in asthma research, laying the foundation for the concept of Th2-driven (T2-high) asthma.

The understanding of asthma phenotypes was further refined by the identification of a subset of patients with severe asthma characterized by airway neutrophilic inflammation [25, 26]. This led to the recognition of neutrophilic asthma (NA), a distinct phenotype with implications for both pathophysiology and treatment. These findings emphasized the importance of airway inflammatory profiles, particularly the presence of eosinophils and/or neutrophils, in defining asthma phenotypes [27, 28].

Since these early developments, respiratory research has identified a broad spectrum of asthma phenotypes, incorporating clinical presentation, physiological and pathological markers, treatment response, and disease prognosis [16].

Several phenotypes have been described for T2-low asthma, such as paucigranulocytic asthma with extensive remodeling, smoking-related asthma, obesity-induced asthma, asthma in the elderly, and post-menopausal asthma [20]. We will further focus on the most common phenotypes of T2-high asthma (**Table 1**).

3.2.1 Early-onset allergic asthma

Early-onset allergic asthma is a well-recognized phenotype of asthma that typically manifests during childhood. It is strongly associated with atopy, a genetic predisposition toward developing allergic hypersensitivity reactions, and is characterized by elevated serum IgE levels, positive skin prick tests, and eosinophilic airway inflammation [29, 30]. This phenotype is among the most common and best-studied forms of asthma, with a clinical course often beginning early in life and frequently associated with other atopic conditions, such as allergic rhinitis and eczema.

The immunopathology of early-onset allergic asthma is driven predominantly by Type 2 (Th2) immune responses. Allergen exposure leads to activation of dendritic cells, which prime naïve T-helper cells toward a Th2 phenotype. Th2 cells secrete cytokines, such as IL-4, IL-5, and IL-13, promoting IgE production by B cells, eosinophil recruitment, and goblet cell hyperplasia [31]. IgE-mediated mast cell degranulation contributes to bronchoconstriction, mucosal edema, and the further amplification of airway inflammation.

Clinically, patients with early-onset allergic asthma present with recurrent wheezing, coughing, chest tightness, and shortness of breath, particularly in response to allergens, such as dust mites, pollen, or pet dander. The diagnosis is supported by a history of atopy, a family history of allergic diseases, positive skin prick or specific IgE tests, and elevated eosinophil counts [1]. Spirometry may demonstrate reversible airway obstruction.

Although early-onset allergic asthma often improves with age, a significant proportion of individuals continue to experience symptoms into adolescence and adulthood. Persistent exposure to allergens, environmental pollutants, and viral infections

Characteristic	Early-onset allergic asthma	Late-onset non-allergic asthma	Aspirin-exacerbated respiratory disease (AERD)
Typical age of onset	Childhood, often <12 years	Adulthood, usually >40 years	Adulthood, typically 30–50 years
Gender predominance	Slightly more common in males in childhood, females later	More common in females	More common in females
Atopy / allergy association	Strong association; positive skin prick tests, high serum IgE	Rarely associated; negative allergy testing	Not typically allergic; may have non-IgE eosinophilia
Triggering factors	Aeroallergens (dust mite, pollen, pets), viral infections	Respiratory infections, irritants, and obesity-related inflammation	NSAIDs (aspirin, ibuprofen), alcohol, irritants
Underlying inflammation	Type 2 (Th2-high) inflammation with eosinophilia	Type 2, but sometimes non-Type 2 (Th2-low), neutrophilic, or mixed inflammation	Type 2 (eosinophilic) inflammation + overproduction of leukotrienes
IgE levels	Elevated	Usually, normal	Usually normal or mildly elevated
Blood/sputum eosinophils	Elevated	Variable (often normal or low)	Elevated
Lung function decline	Variable, may be mild if well controlled	Often progressive, more severe airway remodeling	Progressive decline is common if uncontrolled
Comorbidities	Allergic rhinitis, eczema	Chronic rhinosinusitis (non-polyp), obesity	Chronic rhinosinusitis with nasal polyps (CRSwNP)
Response to inhaled corticosteroids (ICS)	Usually, good	Often poor or partial	Often partial; leukotriene modifiers help
Other treatments	Allergen avoidance, anti-IgE biologics (omalizumab), IL-4/IL-5/IL-13 blockers	Higher ICS doses, macrolides (in some), biologics for the eosinophilic subset	Avoid NSAIDs, leukotriene receptor antagonists, and aspirin desensitization in specialized centers
Prognosis	Good with control	More severe and persistent	Chronic, often severe, high relapse of nasal polyps

Table 1.
Comparative characteristics of severe T2-high asthma phenotypes.

may contribute to airway remodeling and fixed airflow limitation in some patients [32]. The severity and persistence of symptoms are influenced by genetic factors, the burden of allergen exposure, and the presence of comorbid conditions.

3.2.2 Late-onset non-allergic asthma

Late-onset non-allergic asthma is a distinct phenotype that typically emerges in adulthood, often after the age of 40, and is not associated with atopy. Unlike early-onset allergic asthma, it lacks a strong genetic component or IgE-mediated sensitization. Instead, this phenotype is often characterized by persistent symptoms, a poor response to standard asthma therapies, such as inhaled corticosteroids (ICS), and frequent coexistence with comorbidities, such as nasal polyposis and obesity [28, 33].

The pathophysiology of late-onset non-allergic asthma differs significantly from allergic forms of the disease. The T2 immune and inflammatory signature is driven by the involvement of ILC2 cells and eosinophils [20]. Chronic exposure to irritants such as pollutants or occupational agents may also contribute to airway remodeling and inflammation in these patients by the signaling of epithelial surface alarmins.

Patients with late-onset non-allergic asthma frequently present with persistent cough, wheezing, and dyspnea that begin in middle to late adulthood. They often have negative skin prick tests and low serum IgE levels, but higher levels of eosinophilia, distinguishing them from allergic asthma. Diagnosis is based on clinical history, spirometry with reversibility testing, and exclusion of other causes of adult-onset respiratory symptoms [1]. Induced sputum analysis or FeNO testing can help characterize airway inflammation, though these are not always routinely available.

This asthma phenotype tends to be more severe, with a higher degree of airflow obstruction and is less responsive to conventional therapies, including ICS. Frequent exacerbations, reduced lung function, and chronic symptoms are common. Some patients may experience progressive airflow limitation resembling features of COPD. The prognosis varies but often requires long-term management and frequent treatment adjustments (Moore et al., 2010).

Management of late-onset non-allergic asthma can be challenging. High-dose ICS combined with long-acting beta-agonists (LABAs) are typically used, though with limited success in some patients. Management of comorbidities such as sinusitis, gastroesophageal reflux disease (GERD), and obesity is essential for optimizing outcomes. More recently, targeted therapy with anti-IL5 or anti-IL5R agents has demonstrated promising results in the treatment of this asthma phenotype [34, 35].

3.2.3 Aspirin-exacerbated respiratory disease

Aspirin-Exacerbated Respiratory Disease (AERD), also known as Samter's Triad, is a distinct clinical syndrome characterized by the coexistence of asthma, chronic rhinosinusitis with nasal polyposis (CRSwNP), and sensitivity to aspirin and other nonsteroidal anti-inflammatory drugs (NSAIDs) that inhibit cyclooxygenase-1 (COX-1). First described in the early twentieth century, AERD typically develops in adulthood and is associated with more severe and persistent airway inflammation compared to other asthma phenotypes [36, 37].

AERD is not an IgE-mediated allergy, but rather a dysregulation of arachidonic acid metabolism. The inhibition of COX-1 by NSAIDs shifts arachidonic acid metabolism toward the 5-lipoxygenase pathway, resulting in increased production of cysteinyl leukotrienes (CysLTs), potent inflammatory mediators that cause bronchoconstriction, mucus secretion, and eosinophilic inflammation [38]. Additionally, prostaglandin D2 (PGD2), which acts as a chemoattractant for eosinophils and Th2 cells, is overproduced in AERD [39].

Patients with AERD typically present with adult-onset asthma, often severe, accompanied by chronic sinusitis and recurrent nasal polyps. The hallmark of AERD is a respiratory reaction to aspirin or NSAIDs, including bronchospasm, nasal congestion, and rhinorrhea, usually occurring within 30–180 minutes after drug ingestion [40]. Diagnosis is primarily clinical but may be confirmed by an aspirin challenge test under controlled conditions. Elevated urinary leukotriene E4 (uLTE4) levels may support the diagnosis.

AERD is associated with a chronic and often progressive disease course, with high rates of asthma exacerbations, frequent sinus surgeries due to recurrent polyps, and a poor response to standard corticosteroid therapy. The disease burden is typically high, affecting quality of life and requiring multidisciplinary care [41].

Management of AERD includes avoidance of COX-1 inhibiting NSAIDs, pharmacologic treatment with leukotriene receptor antagonists (e.g., montelukast) or 5-lipoxygenase inhibitors (e.g., zileuton), and the use of nasal corticosteroids and biologics targeting Type 2 inflammation (e.g., dupilumab, omalizumab, mepolizumab) [42]. Aspirin desensitization therapy, followed by daily aspirin use, has also been shown to reduce nasal polyp recurrence and improve asthma control in selected patients [43].

4. Inflammatory endotypes in asthma: Eosinophils, neutrophils, and beyond

T2-high asthma is characterized by a dominant Type 2 (T2) immune-inflammatory response driven by both adaptive (Th2 lymphocytes) and innate (ILC2 cells) immunity. This endotype is characterized by the overexpression of T2 cytokines, including IL-4, IL-5, IL-9, and IL-13, as well as prostaglandin D2, and is associated with the presence of eosinophils in both the airway and peripheral blood. The term eosinophilic asthma is often used interchangeably with T2-high asthma and encompasses both allergic and non-allergic forms, accounting for roughly 50% of severe asthma cases [44, 45].

In allergic asthma, exposure to allergens activates dendritic cells, which initiate a Th2 response through the production of cytokines, such as IL-4, resulting in the production of IgE. Cross-linking of allergen-specific IgE on mast cells triggers the release of mediators, such as histamine, leading to bronchoconstriction and inflammation during both the early and late allergic responses [46].

T2 innate immunity is initiated at the epithelial level, where injured bronchial epithelial cells release alarmins—IL-25, IL-33, and TSLP—which further amplify Th2- and ILC2-driven inflammation. These cells release cytokines that recruit and activate eosinophils, induce IgE switching, and contribute to bronchial hyperresponsiveness. IL-4 and IL-13 also stimulate nitric oxide production in the epithelium, measurable as FeNO, a non-invasive biomarker for T2 inflammation [47].

Alongside inflammation, airway remodeling is a hallmark of T2-high asthma. This includes goblet cell metaplasia and mucus plug formation, which are more persistent in severe cases and closely linked to eosinophilic activity [48].

Emerging research also points to a role for exosomal microRNAs in regulating immune responses in T2-high asthma. For instance, increased levels of miR-21-5p and miR-126-3p are associated with Th2 differentiation in atopic phenotypes [49].

Biomarkers such as blood and sputum eosinophils (B-EOS, S-EOS), fractional exhaled nitric oxide (FeNO), and serum total IgE are currently the most validated tools for identifying T2-high asthma phenotypes, predicting disease course, and guiding personalized treatment.

Based on sputum cytology, asthma can be subdivided into four inflammatory endotypes: eosinophilic, neutrophilic, mixed granulocytic, and paucigranulocytic asthma. Eosinophilic asthma, which affects approximately 40–50% of patients, is characterized by elevated eosinophil levels and often responds well to corticosteroids and biologic therapies. It typically aligns with the T2-high endotype and may feature biomarkers, such as blood eosinophils ≥150/μL, FeNO ≥20 ppb, and sputum eosinophils ≥2% (**Figure 1**).

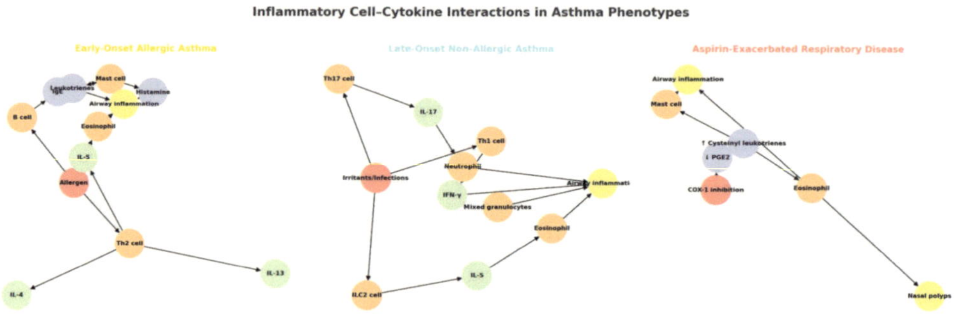

Figure 1.
Inflammatory pathways in severe asthma phenotypes.

Conversely, T2-low asthma, which includes neutrophilic, mixed, and paucigranulocytic subtypes, is less responsive to corticosteroids and often more severe. Neutrophilic asthma, in particular, is frequently associated with smoking, occupational exposures, and chronic infections. It exhibits persistent airway inflammation and poor symptom control despite high-dose inhaled therapies. Patients with mixed granulocytic asthma—elevated eosinophils and neutrophils—present additional therapeutic challenges.

The paucigranulocytic phenotype, characterized by low levels of both eosinophils and neutrophils, remains poorly understood. It may involve non-inflammatory mechanisms, such as airway hyperresponsiveness or neurogenic inflammation, and is often mild but resistant to conventional therapies.

5. Phenotype overlap

The precise characterization of asthma phenotypes is essential for optimizing disease management, as stratifying patients into well-defined clinical subsets facilitates targeted therapeutic interventions. Nonetheless, the inherent heterogeneity of asthma—particularly in its severe forms—frequently gives rise to complex interactions among multiple immunological pathways, resulting in phenotypic overlap and potentially atypical clinical trajectories. Individuals who exhibit a Type 2 (T2) inflammatory profile early in life, especially during infancy, are likely to be exposed to a wide range of environmental factors throughout their lives. These exposures may activate additional immunopathological mechanisms, thereby modulating the initial T2-dominant phenotype and contributing to a more heterogeneous disease presentation [20].

6. Illustrative clinical case reports

6.1 Case report of a late-onset severe eosinophilic asthma super-responder to anti-IL5R therapy

We present a case study based on a 67-year-old patient, an ex-smoker (10 pack years) with long-term exposure to exhaust fumes and biomass fuel, and no evidence of other chronic diseases or allergies, who was diagnosed in the previous year with moderate asthma [50]. The diagnosis was based on fixed moderate obstructive ventilatory dysfunction and significant postbronchodilator reversibility in FEV1. The patient was prescribed an ICS/LABA fixed-dose combination inhaler.

In May 2019, the patient presented with exacerbated symptoms (dyspnea on minimal effort, persistent and productive cough, mucous sputum, intermittent wheezing, serous rhinorrhea, and nocturnal awakenings, ACT score = 14) and was treated with ICS/LABA and oral corticosteroids. Follow-up in June showed improvement, but the condition worsened again by February 2020, leading to higher doses of medication. In April 2020, a severe exacerbation required hospitalization, revealing respiratory failure and cardiovascular issues. Despite high doses of inhaled medication, symptoms persisted, and by July 2020, the patient's condition continued to decline in parallel with a significant rise in blood eosinophil levels of up to 1000 cells/microliter and a constant decline in lung function (lowest FEV1 = 18%). Prednisone was added as maintenance treatment, yet clinical deterioration led to the challenge of debating the diagnosis between asthma (because of high variability of symptoms and functional tests, the good response to ICS/OCS treatment) and COPD (onset age higher than 40 years old, exposure to noxious particles, smoking, persistent airflow limitation). Asthma was diagnosed, excluding parasitic infections and eosinophilic granulomatosis. We mention that the patient had an adequate inhalation technique and a good adherence to the prescribed inhaled medication.

A decision was made to start a biological treatment protocol with benralizumab (30 mg/month for 2 months, then every 2 months). In July 2020, the first dose was administered without adverse reactions. The patient continued high-dose ICS/LABA and 5 mg/day prednisone. The start of benralizumab therapy improved the patient's condition immediately, with no further exacerbations and gradual stepping down of maintenance therapy. After 2 months, the patient's clinical and functional response was very positive (ACT score = 22, FEV1% = 86%), and prednisone was withdrawn. By the third dose, the blood eosinophil level was completely depleted. At the time of publication, the patient reported no asthma exacerbation episodes, total control of typical symptoms (ACT score = 25), spirometry showing mild fixed obstructive ventilatory dysfunction (FEV1% = 116%, FEV1/FVC = 0.64), and maintained a favorable clinical evolution.

This case report discusses benralizumab's efficacy in a patient with a challenging differential diagnosis between asthma and COPD. Despite adequate maintenance treatment, the patient's condition worsened until the initiation of anti-IL5R therapy, which resulted in the achievement of asthma control.

It also highlights an example of late-onset severe eosinophilic asthma refractory to conventional optimized inhaled therapy, in which full remission was achieved with targeted biologic therapy, despite the persistence of mild fixed airway obstruction.

6.2 Case report of a severe allergic asthma patient with recurrent blood eosinophilia

We present another case study [51] based on a 63-year-old female non-smoker with a history of biomass exposure and passive tobacco smoke, who was diagnosed with asthma in 2004, with poor symptom control despite adequate maintenance therapy with Budesonide/Formoterol 320/9 mcg b.i.d. and Montelukast 10 mg o.d., an appropriate inhalation technique, and good compliance.

On 26 November 2018, she experienced a severe exacerbation involving nocturnal non-productive cough, dyspnea, and wheezing, with clear chest X-ray but elevated eosinophils, ESR, and CRP. Spirometry unveiled moderate distal obstructive syndrome. She was prescribed a 7-day course of Prednisone.

On 14 January 2019, another exacerbation episode occurred, with spirometry indicating severe fixed obstruction (FEV1 at 35% with a FEV1/FVC ratio < 0.7) and post-bronchodilator test showing reversibility. Treatment was escalated to Fluticasone/Salmeterol 50/500 mcg b.i.d. and a 10-day Prednisone course; additionally, it was advised that the patient seek consultation with an allergologist for further assessment and management. The test results showed sensitization to dust mites, specifically Dermatophagoides pteronyssinus and farinae. The main recommendation was to reduce dust mite exposure in the patient's home. Additionally, an assessment of total and specific IgE levels was recommended.

On 4 September 2019, an upper respiratory infection triggered an exacerbation episode with cough, mucopurulent exacerbation, dyspnea, low-grade fever, nocturnal awakenings, frequent sneezing, watery rhinorrhea, and wheezing. The ACT score was 16, revealing suboptimal control; additionally, forced spirometry testing revealed moderate obstructive ventilatory impairment, with FEV1 = 64% and FEV1/FVC ratio > 0.7. Antibiotics and symptomatic treatment were administered. Symptoms worsened by 10 September, prompting another Prednisone course.

By 30 October 2019, the patient exhibited persistent cough, dyspnea, and wheezing, with an ACT score still at 16. Functional evaluation showed mild obstruction (FEV1 at 77%), and total IgE was 48.3 IU/mL. The severe asthma diagnosis was confirmed, remaining uncontrolled despite maximal inhaled therapy, good adherence, and proper management of comorbidities, with three exacerbations requiring corticosteroids in the past year.

The patient was initiated on omalizumab (150 mg) and was switched to Beclomethasone/Formoterol (200/6 mcg DPI, 2 inhalations b.i.d.). After 4 months, coughing decreased with no dyspnea or wheezing. The ACT score improved to 23, and spirometry showed mild obstruction (FEV1 at 70%). With positive progress, omalizumab continued alongside adjusted therapy: Beclomethasone/Formoterol 200/6 mcg (1 puff b.i.d.), Montelukast (10 mg o.d.), and Ventolin (100 mcg as needed). Over 12 months, symptom control was maintained without exacerbations. However, after 16 months, the patient started to experience multiple episodes of exacerbations alongside a significant decrease in lung function and a significant rise in blood eosinophil level.

On 21 December 2021, severe eosinophilic asthma was diagnosed, which remained uncontrolled despite GINA step 5 treatment, including a biologic agent, and a switch to a different biologic therapy was considered. The treatment strategy involved the cessation of omalizumab and the start of benralizumab. The other controller medication remained unchanged. The response was positive, with remission of symptoms, improved lung function, and no further exacerbations, allowing for a reduction of ICS doses. Relapsing blood eosinophilia was noted before each administration of anti-IL5R therapy, but asthma control remained stable.

The overlap of inflammatory phenotypes in eosinophilic asthma is a complex and dynamic aspect of asthma pathogenesis. From the treatment perspective, omalizumab and benralizumab, distinct in their mechanisms, exhibit differential effects on blood eosinophilia in the treatment of asthma. Omalizumab, targeting immunoglobulin E (IgE), is used in allergic asthma and can reduce blood eosinophil levels by modulating allergic inflammation, particularly in patients unresponsive to standard therapy. In contrast, benralizumab, designed for severe eosinophilic asthma, induces rapid eosinophil depletion via interleukin-5 receptor alpha (IL-5R), leading to nearly complete reduction in blood eosinophil count [52–55].

We presented a case where a patient, after receiving treatment with omalizumab followed by benralizumab, exhibited persistently elevated levels of blood eosinophils without experiencing exacerbation episodes under anti-IL5R therapy. This case highlights the complexity and variability of asthma presentations, molecular phenotype overlap, and treatment responses. While these medications are effective in managing eosinophilic inflammation when administered separately, exceptions like this emphasize the need for careful monitoring and individualized patient management.

6.3 Case report on overlapping pathogenetic mechanisms in a severe allergic asthma patient

We present the case of a 39-year-old male patient, former smoker (8 P.A.), with a history of childhood-onset allergic asthma and chronic rhinosinusitis, with multiple sensitizations to pollens (grass, cereals), house dust mite, and mold. Around the age of 30 years, his asthma was categorized as severe, as the symptoms were not controlled despite optimized inhaled therapy and antileukotriens, and he experienced multiple episodes of exacerbation requiring systemic corticosteroids. During phenotyping, he presented evidence of T2-high inflammation with a total IgE level of 1379 IU/mL and blood eosinophils of 846 cells/μL.

In 2017, he was initiated on biologic therapy with omalizumab, which was administered for approximately 1.5 years. In March 2019, omalizumab was stopped due to a lack of efficacy. He was administering fluticasone/salmeterol 500/50 mcg b.i.d. inhaled, montelukast 10 mg o.d., levocetirizine 5 mg o.d. orally, and mometasone 50 mcg b.i.d intranasally; however, his asthma was not controlled (ACT score = 16), he experienced repeated exacerbations, and hence, he was put on maintenance oral prednisone (10 mg/day). Spirometry showed severe fixed obstructive dysfunction (FEV1 = 31% predicted), total IgE was 358.3 IU/mL, and blood eosinophils were up to 370 cells/μL. Chest imaging was normal. In June 2020, when benralizumab became available on the local market, the patient was started on this biologic with a good clinical response, good symptom control (ACT score > 20), improved lung function (FEV1 up to 63% predicted), and no exacerbation episodes, which allowed the withdrawal of maintenance prednisone.

The favorable evolution continued for the following 4 years; however, we noticed a constant decline in lung function, the patient continued to experience rhinosinusitis symptoms, asthma symptoms were partially controlled, and he presented an asthma exacerbation episode requiring systemic corticosteroids in 2023. The FeNO test showed a value of 131 ppb in February 2024. Because of this evidence, a decision was made in June 2024 to switch the biologic therapy from benralizumab to dupilumab. Surprisingly, the clinical response was not as expected, with a deterioration of asthma symptom control, recurrence of exacerbation episodes, a decrease in lung function, the need for oral corticosteroids, and a significant rise in blood eosinophils to 3000 cells/μL, which prompted the reinitiation of therapy with an IL5-R agent. The symptom control was again achieved, with no further exacerbations or need for oral corticosteroids; however, the lung function remained poor.

In the age of biologic therapy, achieving remission in severe asthma is no longer a utopia. Despite the excellent efficacy of biologic agents in severe asthmatics, a significant proportion of these patients remain uncontrolled and require long-term oral corticosteroids. Several reasons for this include the presence of multiple overlapping pathogenetic mechanisms that are insufficiently blocked by a single biologic agent, the switching of the molecular phenotype over time, or the development of antibodies against the biologic agent. Currently, there is no clear guidance on how and when to switch between the available biologic agents, and to date, only limited data have been published on the combination of two different biologics; hence, dual therapy is not currently recommended by the existing guidelines.

Child-onset severe allergic asthma typically responds well to biologic therapy with anti-IgE monoclonal antibodies. In our patient, the efficacy of omalizumab was modest, and this therapy was discontinued. Furthermore, the clinical response to anti IL5-R agent was better than expected; however, clinical remission was not achieved. Even more surprisingly, we were able to notice no favorable effect of anti-IL4-R therapy. We believe that the predominance of eosinophilic mechanisms of inflammation in this patient may be explained by past tobacco exposure and/or a possible phenotype switch, while incomplete remission under anti-IL5-R therapy probably indicates an insufficient blocking of all the inflammatory pathways, making this patient a suitable candidate for an anti-TSLP agent, currently not reimbursed in our country and/or dual biologic therapy.

7. Conclusion

Severe asthma is a heterogeneous disease composed of distinct phenotypes and endotypes, each defined by specific clinical and molecular characteristics. While phenotyping offers valuable insights into observable traits, such as age of onset, atopy, and inflammation type, endotyping reveals the underlying immunopathology, particularly by distinguishing between T2-high and T2-low pathways.

T2-high asthma responds well to targeted biologic therapies (e.g., anti-IL-5, anti-IL-4Rα, anti-IgE), whereas T2-low asthma remains less clearly defined and therapeutically challenging. Phenotypic and endotypic overlap—shaped by genetic and environmental factors—further complicates management and underscores the importance of individualized, biomarker-driven approaches.

Advancing our understanding of these complex mechanisms is key to optimizing treatment and improving outcomes in patients with severe asthma.

Acknowledgements

I would like to acknowledge VICTOR BABES UNIVERSITY OF MEDICINE AND PHARMACY TIMISOARA for their support in covering the costs of publication of this book chapter.

Conflict of interest

The author declares no conflict of interest.

Author details

Stefan-Marian Frent
Center for Research and Innovation in Precision Medicine of Respiratory Diseases, Department of Pulmonology, "Victor Babes" University of Medicine and Pharmacy Timisoara, Timisoara, Romania

*Address all correspondence to: frentz.stefan@umft.ro

References

[1] Global Initiative for Asthma (GINA). Global Strategy for Asthma Management and Prevention. 2025. Available from: https://ginasthma.org/2025-gina-strategy-report [Accessed: July 02, 2025]

[2] Busse WW. Biological treatments for severe asthma: A major advance in asthma care. Allergology International. 2019;**68**(2):158-166. DOI: 10.1016/j.alit.2019.01.004

[3] Barnes PJ. Pathophysiology of asthma. British Journal of Clinical Pharmacology. Jul 1996;**42**(1):3-10. DOI: 10.1046/j.1365-2125.1996.03721.x

[4] Gauvreau GM, Sehmi R, Ambrose CS, Griffiths JM. Thymic stromal lymphopoietin: Its role and potential as a therapeutic target in asthma. Expert Opinion on Therapeutic Targets. 2020;**24**(8):777-792. DOI: 10.1080/14728222.2020.178324

[5] Berair R, Hollins F, Brightling C. Airway smooth muscle hypercontractility in asthma. Journal of Allergy (Cairo). 2013;**2013**:185971. DOI: 10.1155/2013/185971

[6] Chapman DG, Irvin CG. Mechanisms of airway hyper-responsiveness in asthma: The past, present and yet to come. Clinical and Experimental Allergy. 2015;**45**(4):706-719. DOI: 10.1111/cea.12506

[7] Chung KF, Wenzel SE, Brozek JL, Bush A, Castro M, Sterk PJ, et al. International ERS/ATS guidelines on definition, evaluation and treatment of severe asthma. The European Respiratory Journal. 2014;**43**(2):343-373. DOI: 10.1183/09031936.00202013

[8] Wenzel S. Severe asthma: From characteristics to phenotypes to endotypes. Clinical and Experimental Allergy. 2012;**42**(5):650-658. DOI: 10.1111/j.1365-2222.2011.03929.x

[9] Fitzpatrick AM, Moore WC. Severe asthma phenotypes - How should they guide evaluation and treatment? The Journal of Allergy and Clinical Immunology. In Practice. 2017;**5**(4):901-908. DOI: 10.1016/j.jaip.2017.05.015

[10] Pavord ID, Beasley R, Agusti A, Anderson GP, Bel E, Brusselle G, et al. After asthma: Redefining airways diseases. Lancet. 2018;**391**(10118):350-400. DOI: 10.1016/S0140-6736(17)30879-6

[11] Barnes PJ. Targeting cytokines to treat asthma and chronic obstructive pulmonary disease. Nature Reviews. Immunology. 2018;**18**(7):454-466. DOI: 10.1038/s41577-018-0006-6

[12] Plosker GL, Keam SJ. Omalizumab: A review of its use in the treatment of allergic asthma. BioDrugs. 2008;**22**(3):189-204. DOI: 10.2165/00063030-200822030-00005

[13] Castro M, Corren J, Pavord ID, Maspero J, Wenzel S, Rabe KF, et al. Dupilumab efficacy and safety in moderate-to-severe uncontrolled asthma. The New England Journal of Medicine. 2018;**378**(26):2486-2496. DOI: 10.1056/NEJMoa1804092

[14] Menzies-Gow A, Corren J, Bourdin A, Chupp G, Israel E, Wechsler ME, et al. Tezepelumab in adults and adolescents with severe, uncontrolled asthma. The New England Journal of Medicine. 2021;**384**(19):1800-1809. DOI: 10.1056/NEJMoa2034975

[15] Cunha F, Amaral R, Jacinto T, Sousa-Pinto B, Fonseca JA. A systematic review of asthma phenotypes derived by data-driven methods. Diagnostics (Basel). 2021;**11**(4):644. DOI: 10.3390/diagnostics11040644

[16] Agache I, Akdis C, Jutel M, Virchow JC. Untangling asthma phenotypes and endotypes. Allergy. 2012;**67**(7):835-846. DOI: 10.1111/j.1398-9995.2012.02832.x

[17] Lötvall J, Akdis CA, Bacharier LB, Bjermer L, Casale TB, Custovic A, et al. Asthma endotypes: A new approach to classification of disease entities within the asthma syndrome. The Journal of Allergy and Clinical Immunology. 2011;**127**(2):355-360. DOI: 10.1016/j.jaci.2010.11.037

[18] Anderson GP. Endotyping asthma: New insights into key pathogenic mechanisms in a complex, heterogeneous disease. Lancet. 2008;**372**(9643):1107-1119. DOI: 10.1016/S0140-6736(08)61452-X

[19] Brasier AR, Victor S, Boetticher G, Ju H, Lee C, Bleecker ER, et al. Molecular phenotyping of severe asthma using pattern recognition of bronchoalveolar lavage-derived cytokines. The Journal of Allergy and Clinical Immunology. 2008;**121**(1):30-37.e6. DOI: 10.1016/j.jaci.2007.10.015

[20] Ricciardolo FLM, Guida G, Bertolini F, Di Stefano A, Carriero V. Phenotype overlap in the natural history of asthma. European Respiratory Review. 2023;**32**(168):220201. DOI: 10.1183/16000617.0201-2022

[21] Rackemann FM. A working classification of asthma. The American Journal of Medicine. 1947;**3**(5):601-606. DOI: 10.1016/0002-9343(47)90204-0

[22] Bentley AM, Menz G, Storz C, Robinson DS, Bradley B, Jeffery PK, et al. Identification of T lymphocytes, macrophages, and activated eosinophils in the bronchial mucosa in intrinsic asthma. Relationship to symptoms and bronchial responsiveness. The American Review of Respiratory Disease. 1992;**146**(2):500-506. DOI: 10.1164/ajrccm/146.2.500

[23] Humbert M, Menz G, Ying S, Corrigan CJ, Robinson DS, Durham SR, et al. The immunopathology of extrinsic (atopic) and intrinsic (non-atopic) asthma: More similarities than differences. Immunology Today. 1999;**20**(11):528-533. DOI: 10.1016/s0167-5699(99)01535-2

[24] Robinson DS, Hamid Q, Ying S, Tsicopoulos A, Barkans J, Bentley AM, et al. Predominant TH2-like bronchoalveolar T-lymphocyte population in atopic asthma. The New England Journal of Medicine. 1992;**326**(5):298-304. DOI: 10.1056/NEJM199201303260504

[25] The ENFUMOSA cross-sectional European multicentre study of the clinical phenotype of chronic severe asthma. European Network for Understanding Mechanisms of Severe Asthma. The European Respiratory Journal. 2003;**22**(3):470-477. DOI: 10.1183/09031936.03.00261903

[26] Wenzel SE, Schwartz LB, Langmack EL, Halliday JL, Trudeau JB, Gibbs RL, et al. Evidence that severe asthma can be divided pathologically into two inflammatory subtypes with distinct physiologic and clinical characteristics. American Journal of Respiratory and Critical Care Medicine. 1999;**160**(3):1001-1008. DOI: 10.1164/ajrccm.160.3.9812110

[27] Wenzel SE. Asthma: Defining of the persistent adult phenotypes. Lancet.

2006;**368**(9537):804-813. DOI: 10.1016/S0140-6736(06)69290-8

[28] Wenzel SE. Asthma phenotypes: The evolution from clinical to molecular approaches. Nature Medicine. 2012;**18**(5):716-725. DOI: 10.1038/nm.2678

[29] Martinez FD, Wright AL, Taussig LM, Holberg CJ, Halonen M, Morgan WJ. Asthma and wheezing in the first six years of life. The Group Health Medical Associates. The New England Journal of Medicine. 1995;**332**(3):133-138. DOI: 10.1056/NEJM199501193320301

[30] Custovic A, Simpson A. The role of inhalant allergens in allergic airways disease. Journal of Investigational Allergology & Clinical Immunology. 2012;**22**(6):393-401 qiuz follow 401

[31] Holgate ST. Innate and adaptive immune responses in asthma. Nature Medicine. 2012;**18**(5):673-683. DOI: 10.1038/nm.2731

[32] Lange P, Parner J, Vestbo J, Schnohr P, Jensen G. A 15-year follow-up study of ventilatory function in adults with asthma. The New England Journal of Medicine. 1998;**339**(17):1194-1200. DOI: 10.1056/NEJM199810223391703

[33] Haldar P, Pavord ID, Shaw DE, Berry MA, Thomas M, Brightling CE, et al. Cluster analysis and clinical asthma phenotypes. American Journal of Respiratory and Critical Care Medicine. 2008;**178**(3):218-224. DOI: 10.1164/rccm.200711-1754OC

[34] Prazma CM, Idzko M, Douglass JA, Bourdin A, Mallett S, Albers FC, et al. Response to mepolizumab treatment in patients with severe eosinophilic asthma and atopic phenotypes. Journal of Asthma and Allergy. 2021;**14**:675-683. DOI: 10.2147/JAA.S298559

[35] Chia YL, Yan L, Yu B, Wang B, Barker P, Goldman M, et al. Relationship between benralizumab exposure and efficacy for patients with severe eosinophilic asthma. Clinical Pharmacology and Therapeutics. 2019;**106**(2):383-390. DOI: 10.1002/cpt.1371

[36] Stevenson DD, Szczeklik A. Clinical and pathologic perspectives on aspirin sensitivity and asthma. The Journal of Allergy and Clinical Immunology. Oct 2006;**118**(4):773-786; quiz 787-8. DOI: 10.1016/j.jaci.2006.07.024

[37] Cahill KN, Bensko JC, Boyce JA, Laidlaw TM. Prostaglandin D_2: A dominant mediator of aspirin-exacerbated respiratory disease. The Journal of Allergy and Clinical Immunology. 2015;**135**(1):245-252. DOI: 10.1016/j.jaci.2014.07.031

[38] Laidlaw TM, Boyce JA. Aspirin-exacerbated respiratory disease–new prime suspects. The New England Journal of Medicine. 2016;**374**(5):484-488. DOI: 10.1056/NEJMcibr1514013

[39] Steinke JW, Wilson JM. Aspirin-exacerbated respiratory disease: Pathophysiological insights and clinical advances. Journal of Asthma and Allergy. 2016;**9**:37-43. DOI: 10.2147/JAA.S88739

[40] White AA, Stevenson DD. Aspirin-exacerbated respiratory disease. The New England Journal of Medicine. 2018;**379**(11):1060-1070. DOI: 10.1056/NEJMra1712125

[41] Shah SA, Kobayashi M. Pathogenesis of chronic rhinosinusitis with nasal polyp and a prominent T2 endotype. Heliyon. 2023;**9**(9):e19249. DOI: 10.1016/j.heliyon.2023.e19249

[42] Hayashi H, Ishii M, Hasegawa Y, Taniguchi M. Critical pathomechanisms

of NSAID-exacerbated respiratory disease (N-ERD) clarified by treatment with omalizumab, an anti-IgE antibody. Allergology International. 2025;**74**(1):51-65. DOI: 10.1016/j.alit.2024.08.008

[43] Lee RU, Stevenson DD. Aspirin-exacerbated respiratory disease: Evaluation and management. Allergy, Asthma & Immunology Research. 2011;**3**(1):3-10. DOI: 10.4168/aair.2011.3.1.3

[44] Kaur R, Chupp G. Phenotypes and endotypes of adult asthma: Moving toward precision medicine. The Journal of Allergy and Clinical Immunology. 2019;**144**(1):1-12. DOI: 10.1016/j.jaci.2019.05.031

[45] Zervas E, Samitas K, Papaioannou AI, Bakakos P, Loukides S, Gaga M. An algorithmic approach for the treatment of severe uncontrolled asthma. ERJ Open Research. 2018;**4**(1):00125-02017. DOI: 10.1183/23120541.00125-2017

[46] Lambrecht BN, Hammad H. The airway epithelium in asthma. Nature Medicine. 2012;**18**(5):684-692. DOI: 10.1038/nm.2737

[47] Ricciardolo FLM, Silkoff PE. Perspectives on exhaled nitric oxide. Journal of Breath Research. 2017;**11**(4):047104. DOI: 10.1088/1752-7163/aa7f0e

[48] Dunican EM, Elicker BM, Gierada DS, Nagle SK, Schiebler ML, Newell JD, et al. Mucus plugs in patients with asthma linked to eosinophilia and airflow obstruction. The Journal of Clinical Investigation. 2018;**128**(3):997-1009. DOI: 10.1172/JCI95693

[49] Vázquez-Mera S, Martelo-Vidal L, Miguéns-Suárez P, Saavedra-Nieves P, Arias P, González-Fernández C, et al. Serum exosome inflamma-miRs are surrogate biomarkers for asthma phenotype and severity. Allergy. 2023;**78**(1):141-155. DOI: 10.1111/all.15480

[50] Oprescu B, Raduna O, Mihaicuta S, Frent S. Severe asthma or chronic obstructive pulmonary disease with eosinophilic inflammation? From uncertainty to remission under anti IL-5R therapy. Medicina (Kaunas, Lithuania). 2024;**60**(3):387. DOI: 10.3390/medicina60030387

[51] Raduna O, Oprescu B, Mihaicuta S, Frent S. Relapsing eosinophilia in a severe allergic asthma patient on biological therapy. Journal of Clinical Medicine. 2024;**13**(12):3402. DOI: 10.3390/jcm13123402

[52] Hanania NA, Wenzel S, Rosén K, Hsieh HJ, Mosesova S, Choy DF, et al. Exploring the effects of omalizumab in allergic asthma: An analysis of biomarkers in the EXTRA study. American Journal of Respiratory and Critical Care Medicine. 2013;**187**(8):804-811. DOI: 10.1164/rccm.201208-1414OC

[53] Corren J, Casale TB, Lanier B, Buhl R, Holgate S, Jimenez P. Safety and tolerability of omalizumab. Clinical and Experimental Allergy. 2009;**39**(6):788-797. DOI: 10.1111/j.1365-2222.2009.03214.x

[54] Bleecker ER, FitzGerald JM, Chanez P, Papi A, Weinstein SF, Barker P, et al. Efficacy and safety of benralizumab for patients with severe asthma uncontrolled with high-dosage inhaled corticosteroids and long-acting β_2-agonists (SIROCCO): A randomised, multicentre, placebo-controlled phase 3 trial. Lancet. 2016;**388**(10056):2115-2127. DOI: 10.1016/S0140-6736(16)31324-1

[55] FitzGerald JM, Bleecker ER, Nair P, Korn S, Ohta K, Lommatzsch M,

et al. CALIMA study investigators. Benralizumab, an anti-interleukin-5 receptor α monoclonal antibody, as add-on treatment for patients with severe, uncontrolled, eosinophilic asthma (CALIMA): A randomised, double-blind, placebo-controlled phase 3 trial. Lancet. 2016;**388**(10056):2128-2141. DOI: 10.1016/S0140-6736(16)31322-8

Chapter 6

The Effect of Asthma Exacerbations on Pregnancy Outcomes

Nasrin Fazel

Abstract

Asthma exacerbations during pregnancy remain understudied, and their impact on pregnancy outcomes is not well understood. This prospective cohort study examined 34 pregnant women with asthma, assessing exacerbation severity and asthma control throughout pregnancy. Findings revealed that more than half of women with intermittent or mild asthma and a smaller proportion of those with moderate or severe asthma experienced severe exacerbations. Nearly half of the participants had worsened asthma control in the second and third trimesters. Exacerbation severity varied based on place of residence, while maternal age, lung function, body mass index, gravidity, and parity showed no clear influence. Seasonal patterns emerged, with the highest number of exacerbations occurring in winter. Exposure to allergens, such as dust, pollen, and smoke, was associated with pregnancy complications, including bleeding, pain before delivery, and urinary tract infections. The high rate of exacerbations among pregnant women with asthma highlights the need for effective management strategies to reduce complications and ensure the well-being of both mother and fetus.

Keywords: asthma, exacerbations, pregnancy, allergen, perinatal outcomes

1. Introduction

Asthma is a prevalent chronic respiratory condition that affects a significant percentage of pregnant women, with estimates ranging between 3 and 12% globally [1].

2. Pathophysiology of asthma in pregnancy

2.1 Mechanisms of asthma

The physiological changes that occur during pregnancy can influence asthma severity, potentially leading to an increased risk of exacerbations [2]. Managing asthma in pregnant women poses a unique challenge due to concerns about medication safety and its impact on fetal development. Research has shown that inadequate asthma control can lead to adverse maternal and fetal outcomes, including preterm birth, low birth weight, and increased neonatal morbidity [3]. However, evidence regarding the exact mechanisms linking asthma exacerbations to perinatal outcomes remains inconclusive [4].

During pregnancy, hormonal changes, such as increased progesterone levels and alterations in immune function, can influence respiratory function, which may exacerbate asthma symptoms [5].

2.2 The link between allergies and asthma

Furthermore, respiratory infections, environmental allergens, and non-adherence to asthma medication contribute to worsening asthma control in pregnancy [6]. Studies suggest that asthma symptoms tend to worsen in approximately one-third of pregnant women, remain stable in another third, and improve in the remaining third [7]. However, the mechanisms behind these variations remain poorly understood.

Asthma control in pregnancy is crucial because exacerbations can lead to significant maternal and fetal complications. Poorly managed asthma has been linked to increased risks of hypertensive disorders of pregnancy, cesarean delivery, fetal growth restriction, and neonatal intensive care unit (NICU) admissions [8]. International guidelines recommend continuing asthma medication during pregnancy to maintain disease control, but adherence to treatment remains a significant challenge due to fears regarding medication safety [9].

This review evaluates the findings of *The Effect of Asthma Exacerbation on Pregnancy Outcomes* in the context of allergology and clinical practice. The study's objectives include assessing the prevalence of exacerbations, identifying associated risk factors, and determining their impact on maternal and neonatal health. The findings provide critical insights into the importance of optimizing asthma management during pregnancy and highlight key areas for future research.

2.3 Summary of key findings

The study was a prospective cohort analysis conducted at Mobini Hospital, Iran, involving 1603 pregnant women, of whom 34 were identified as asthmatic. The investigation focused on the frequency of asthma exacerbations, associated risk factors, and their impact on maternal and fetal outcomes.

3. Asthma exacerbations and their impact on pregnancy

3.1 Exacerbation prevalence and risk factors

As many as 53.1% of women with mild or intermittent asthma experienced exacerbations, whereas 12.5% of those with moderate to severe asthma reported exacerbations [10]. The primary triggers for exacerbations included viral infections, non-adherence to inhaled corticosteroid therapy, and allergen exposure [11]. Maternal cold, smoking exposure, and urban residency were significantly associated with higher exacerbation rates [12].

3.2 Maternal and neonatal outcomes

Severe exacerbations were linked to a higher incidence of maternal complications, including urinary tract infections (UTIs), pregnancy-induced hypertension (PIH), and vaginal bleeding [13]. No statistically significant differences were observed in neonatal birth weight or gestational age between those who experienced exacerbations and those who did not [14]. Allergic reactions were significantly associated with increased pre-labor pain and UTIs [15].

3.3 Asthma medication and control

The study found that 92.6% of asthmatic pregnant women were on routine medication, including inhaled corticosteroids (ICS) and long-acting beta-agonists (LABA) [16]. Women who adhered to their asthma management regimen experienced fewer severe exacerbations, reinforcing the importance of continued medication use during pregnancy [17].

3.4 Maternal and neonatal outcomes

Asthma exacerbations during pregnancy can significantly impact maternal health and fetal development, with varying degrees of severity depending on the frequency and intensity of exacerbations.

3.4.1 Maternal outcomes

Women who experienced severe asthma exacerbations were found to be at increased risk of pregnancy complications, including:

- *Pregnancy-induced hypertension (PIH)*: Several studies have reported an association between uncontrolled asthma and hypertensive disorders in pregnancy, possibly due to systemic inflammation and vascular dysfunction.

- *Gestational diabetes mellitus (GDM)*: While data are inconclusive, some findings suggest that inflammation and altered immune responses in asthmatic women may contribute to glucose metabolism disturbances.

- *Urinary tract infections (UTIs)*: Women with frequent exacerbations were more likely to develop UTIs, potentially due to immunological changes and increased inflammation.

- *Preterm labor and pre-labor pain*: A higher incidence of pre-labor pain and contractions was noted among women with poorly controlled asthma, possibly linked to immune activation and increased uterine irritability.

- *Vaginal bleeding*: Increased episodes of vaginal bleeding, especially in later pregnancy stages, were observed in women with asthma exacerbations, which may be associated with inflammation and endothelial dysfunction.

- *Cesarean delivery (C-section) risk*: Women with severe exacerbations had a slightly higher likelihood of requiring a C-section, possibly due to fetal distress or maternal complications.

Despite these risks, the study found no statistically significant differences in maternal weight gain, body mass index (BMI), or parity between women with and without severe exacerbations.

3.4.2 Neonatal outcomes

The effects of asthma exacerbations on neonatal health remain complex, with mixed findings in the literature. Key neonatal outcomes examined in this study include:

- *Birth weight and fetal growth*: No statistically significant differences were observed in neonatal birth weight between infants born to mothers with and without exacerbations. However, previous studies have reported a potential association between severe exacerbations and fetal growth restriction.

- *Preterm birth*: While a slightly increased rate of preterm birth was noted among women with severe exacerbations, the difference was not statistically significant.

- *Neonatal intensive care unit (NICU) admissions*: Infants born to mothers who had exacerbations had a marginally higher NICU admission rate, though not at a statistically significant level. This may be attributed to transient respiratory distress rather than structural anomalies.

- *Congenital anomalies*: No clear association was found between asthma exacerbations and congenital anomalies, consistent with previous research. However, certain studies suggest that maternal asthma control, rather than exacerbations alone, may influence fetal development.

- *Apgar scores*: Most infants born to mothers with asthma exacerbations had normal Apgar scores at birth, suggesting minimal immediate impact on neonatal adaptation.

3.4.3 Influence of medication adherence

Medication adherence played a significant role in maternal and neonatal outcomes:

- *Women who adhered to inhaled corticosteroid (ICS) therapy experienced fewer severe exacerbations* and had better overall pregnancy outcomes.

- *Non-adherence to asthma medication was linked to more frequent exacerbations and increased risk of pregnancy complications.*

These findings reinforce the importance of continued asthma management during pregnancy to prevent exacerbations and reduce the risk of maternal and neonatal complications.

4. Management of asthma during pregnancy

Among the 1603 pregnant women in the study, 34 were diagnosed with asthma. Severe exacerbations occurred in a small percentage of these women during pregnancy, while mild exacerbations were more common. The frequency of worsening asthma control and exacerbations increased as pregnancy progressed, with a notable proportion occurring in the third trimester.

Women who experienced severe asthma exacerbations were more likely to have a normal body mass index rather than being underweight. The majority of asthmatic pregnant women were of Turkish descent. Most of them received routine asthma treatment, including long-acting β2-agonists, while a small proportion did not take any medication during pregnancy. Nearly all asthmatic women were non-smokers. A few women did not use inhaled corticosteroids at any time during pregnancy.

When comparing women who experienced severe exacerbations with those who did not, no major differences were found in terms of maternal age, education, height, weight, body mass index, gravidity, parity, asthma control, smoking status, or lung function. However, a difference was observed based on place of residence, with urban and rural environments influencing asthma severity.

5. Asthma severity and exacerbation frequency

Asthma severity plays a critical role in determining the frequency and intensity of exacerbations during pregnancy. Women in this study were categorized according to their baseline asthma severity as having *intermittent, mild, moderate, or severe asthma*. The findings indicate that *exacerbation rates varied based on asthma severity*, with women in the *moderate and severe asthma groups* being more susceptible to worsening symptoms and requiring medical intervention.

5.1 Distribution of exacerbations by asthma severity

- *Intermittent and mild asthma*:

  The majority of women in these categories either did not experience exacerbations or had only mild episodes.
  Some women with mild asthma had moderate exacerbations, particularly in the second and third trimesters.
  Adherence to *inhaled corticosteroids (ICS)* and proper asthma management were associated with fewer exacerbations in this group.

- *Moderate and severe asthma*:

  A greater proportion of women with moderate or severe asthma experienced *at least one exacerbation* during pregnancy.
  Severe exacerbations requiring medical intervention were more common in these groups, though *not all women with severe asthma experienced exacerbations*.
  Women in this category showed *higher rates of nocturnal asthma symptoms, increased use of rescue medication, and worsened lung function* compared to those with mild asthma.
  These findings suggest that *while asthma severity is a key factor, not all women with severe asthma experience exacerbations*, highlighting the importance of *individualized asthma management strategies* during pregnancy.

5.2 Healthcare utilization patterns

The frequency and severity of asthma exacerbations influenced healthcare utilization among pregnant women, with *variable patterns based on asthma severity*:

- *Unscheduled doctor visits*:

  Women with *moderate and severe asthma were more likely to seek unplanned medical care* due to worsening symptoms.
  Common reasons for these visits included *shortness of breath, wheezing, and concerns about fetal well-being*.

- *Emergency room (ER) and hospital admissions*:

  A *higher proportion of women with severe asthma required hospitalization* for acute exacerbations compared to those with mild asthma.
  Oral corticosteroid use was more frequent among hospitalized women, indicating a greater need for systemic anti-inflammatory treatment.

- *Use of rescue medication (short-acting beta-agonists—SABA)*:

  Women with severe asthma had *significantly higher usage of rescue inhalers*, reflecting poorer baseline asthma control.
  Frequent SABA use was also linked to *increased likelihood of exacerbations*, reinforcing the importance of maintenance therapy.

- *Oral corticosteroid use*:

  A subset of women, particularly those with moderate to severe asthma, required *oral corticosteroids for exacerbation management*.
  Long-term use of systemic corticosteroids was *avoided when possible*, due to concerns about fetal effects.
  Despite these differences, *the overall patterns of healthcare use were not substantially different between asthma severity groups*, suggesting that factors beyond baseline severity—such as *medication adherence, environmental triggers, and access to care*—also play a role in exacerbation risk.

5.3 Seasonal variation in exacerbations

Seasonal trends in asthma exacerbations were observed, with *the highest number occurring in winter, followed by spring, summer, and autumn*. Potential contributing factors include:

- *Increased respiratory infections (e.g., viral colds, influenza) during winter*, which can trigger exacerbations.

- *Higher indoor allergen exposure in colder months* (e.g., dust mites, mold, pet dander) due to increased time spent indoors.

- *Springtime pollen exposure*, leading to allergy-induced exacerbations in sensitized individuals.

These findings suggest that *seasonal asthma management strategies should be integrated into prenatal care*, particularly during high-risk months.

5.4 Impact of asthma severity on pregnancy outcomes

While severe asthma was associated with a *higher frequency of exacerbations*, the impact on pregnancy outcomes varied:

- Women with well-controlled *severe asthma had pregnancy outcomes comparable to those with mild asthma*, highlighting the importance of effective management.
- Poorly controlled asthma—regardless of baseline severity—was associated with *higher risks of preterm labor, vaginal bleeding, and maternal infections*.
- No significant differences in *birth weight or neonatal complications* were observed between severity groups, though severe exacerbations were linked to a *slightly higher NICU admission rate*.

These results emphasize that *while asthma severity influences exacerbation risk, proper management can mitigate adverse pregnancy outcomes*.

6. Perinatal outcomes in asthmatic pregnant women

Pregnancy outcomes were similar between women who had severe asthma exacerbations and those who did not. Birth weight did not show a clear trend in relation to exacerbations, and the likelihood of delivering a male or female infant was comparable between the two groups. Severe exacerbations did not have a noticeable impact on maternal weight gain during pregnancy. The rate of preterm birth was also similar between the groups, with most women delivering at term.

More than half of the severe exacerbations were associated with maternal cold or upper respiratory tract infections. Seasonal patterns were observed, with the highest number of exacerbations occurring in winter, followed by spring, summer, and autumn.

6.1 Maternal outcomes—Complications in pregnant women with asthma

Women with asthma exacerbations had a higher incidence of urinary tract infections (UTIs), possibly due to inflammation and immune system changes. A significantly higher prevalence of pregnancy-induced hypertension (PIH) was noted among women with severe asthma exacerbations. Vaginal bleeding is observed at a higher rate in women with asthma exacerbations, particularly in the later stages of pregnancy. Increased frequency of pre-labor pain was noted, especially among women with a history of allergic reactions.

6.2 Neonatal outcomes—Birth outcomes in infants born to asthmatic mothers

No statistically significant differences in neonatal birth weight were found between women who had exacerbations and those who did not [9]. A slightly higher likelihood of NICU admission was observed in infants born to mothers with asthma exacerbations, though this was not statistically significant.

No increased risk of congenital anomalies was detected in neonates born to mothers with asthma exacerbations.

7. Impact of environmental and allergenic factors

Asthma exacerbations during pregnancy were influenced by environmental and allergenic factors. While maternal cold or flu symptoms were not strongly linked to birth complications, exposure to allergens, such as dust, pollen, pet dander, smoke, perfumes, and certain foods, appeared to play a role in pregnancy-related complications. Women with higher exposure to these allergens were more likely to experience bleeding, pain before delivery, and urinary tract infections.

Immune system markers, including maternal and infant immunoglobulin E (IgE) levels and eosinophil counts, were also examined. These findings suggest that allergic responses and immune activity may contribute to asthma exacerbations and their effects on pregnancy.

8. Discussion

The exacerbation rate among pregnant women with asthma is high. The study found that 12.5% of women had a severe exacerbation and 53.1% had a mild exacerbation during pregnancy, which align with findings from previous research [10]. However, a notable difference was that the prevalence of severe exacerbations in this study was lower than those reported by Murphy et al. (36%) and Schatz et al. (20%) [16, 17]. These discrepancies may be attributed to differences in asthma classification, medication adherence, and study populations.

The study's results highlight the importance of consistent asthma management to prevent exacerbations. A significant proportion of women with mild asthma who used ICS did not experience severe exacerbations, which is consistent with findings by Murphy et al. [15]. This underscores the necessity of educating pregnant women about the benefits of continued medication use. Previous studies have shown that concerns about medication safety often lead to discontinuation, which increases the risk of uncontrolled asthma and exacerbations [9].

Another key finding was the impact of allergen exposure on pregnancy outcomes. Women who were exposed to allergens had significantly higher risks of UTIs, prelabor pain, and vaginal bleeding [18]. This supports the hypothesis that allergic inflammation plays a role in pregnancy complications. Research suggests that eosinophilic inflammation triggered by allergens may contribute to uterine contractions and preterm labor [19].

Ethnic disparities in exacerbation rates were also observed. Turkish women had higher rates of severe exacerbations compared to Farsi women, a finding that aligns with those of previous studies on asthma disparities in different ethnic populations [20]. Socioeconomic factors, healthcare access, and genetic predispositions may contribute to these differences. Further research is needed to explore the underlying mechanisms behind these disparities and to develop targeted interventions.

9. Clinical implications for allergology and obstetric care

- *Optimizing asthma control*: The findings emphasize that stable asthma control throughout pregnancy is essential for minimizing exacerbations. Asthma treatment guidelines should reinforce adherence to prescribed medications, especially inhaled corticosteroids.

- *Addressing allergen exposure*: Given the observed link between allergen sensitivity and pregnancy complications, allergists and obstetricians should advocate for comprehensive allergen avoidance strategies for pregnant asthmatics.

- *Education and prenatal counseling*: Pregnant women with asthma require targeted education on the risks associated with exacerbations, the safety of asthma medications, and the importance of regular pulmonary function monitoring.

The exacerbation rate among pregnant women with asthma is high. In this study, we found that 12.5% of women had a severe exacerbation and 53.1% of women had a mild exacerbation during pregnancy. We also stratified our subjects by background asthma severity and found a decrease in exacerbation events with increasing asthma severity, as against those previously reported by Murphy et al. Overall, the rate of severe exacerbation (12.5%) was less than that reported by Murphy et al. (36%) [10] but very similar to that reported by Schatz et al. (20%). The classification systems for asthma severity and exacerbations used by Schatz et al. and our study were very similar [13] and the rate among severe asthmatics was also considerably lower (12.5%) compared with those reported by Murphy et al. and Schatz et al., 65 and 52%, respectively [10]. However, in our study some women with mild asthma who used asthma medications (e.g., ICS) had no severe exacerbation results similar to those in Murphy et al.'s study, although in the study from Schatz et al., women with mild asthma used no daily asthma medications [10, 13]. In addition, the proportions of women with mild and severe asthma were quite different between the studies. In our study, 36% of mild and severe asthmatic women did not use asthma drugs, whereas in Schatz et al.'s study, 50% of the women had mild asthma (no medication use) and only 3% of women had severe asthma [13]). Also in Murphy et al.'s study, 36% of women did not use inhaled steroids [10]. This may explain the higher rate of exacerbation found in their study. We had recorded 66.7% asthma attack three times or more in pregnant women with severe asthma. More education is required to inform women that a severe asthma attack presents more of a risk to the fetus than the use of asthma medications because of the potential for a reduction in the supply of oxygen to the fetus [10, 14]. We compared pregnancy outcomes in women who had a severe exacerbation of asthma during pregnancy and those who had no severe exacerbation. Overall, there were no significant trends towards an adverse perinatal outcome due to exacerbations. We had no infants with a birth weight under 2500 g in our severe exacerbation cohort. As well, the neonate's gender has been unaffected by asthma exacerbation, whereas Murphy et al. showed that the mean birth weight of male neonates was approximately 300 g lower when mothers had a severe exacerbation of asthma during pregnancy. The possible explanation of our finding is that the effects of exacerbations during pregnancy are not sex-specific and may be explained by the confounding effect of reduced birth weight in female neonates when mothers used or did not use inhaled steroids, avoiding an exacerbation [10, 15]. Among the hypotheses put forward to explain the mechanisms behind the association between fetal gender and maternal asthma control during pregnancy, the one related to the regulation of placental glucocorticoid and immune response in asthmatic pregnancies seems the most plausible [6]. However, further studies with larger sample sizes should be conducted to investigate these possibilities. We examined our data separately for the known confounding effect of the most common allergens: common cold, allergy, and smoke, and we found that the presence of an allergy in asthmatic women carried the highest risk for bleeding, pain 3 weeks before delivery, and UTI. A prospective cohort study of 101 pregnant women with asthma and 77 control women found that 35% of the asthmatics had a urinary or upper respiratory tract infection compared with only 5% of non-asthmatic women [16]. Most exacerbations were due to viral infections, irrespective of the background inflammatory phenotype, suggesting an altered physiological response to viral infection. It is hypothesized that changes in the maternal immune system, rather than differences in frequency of viral infections, are the cause. During pregnancy, more attention needs to be paid to asthma control and risk of exacerbations [9, 10]. An allergic-like mechanism was proposed as a potential etiology for the preterm parturition syndrome, based on the observation that eosinophils were present in the amniotic fluid in a fraction of women with preterm labor and a history of allergy. Roberto Romero reported an allergic reaction and regular uterine contractions after the ingestion of lobster meat to which the subject was known to be allergic [17]. This probably accounts for the significant relationship between allergy and prolonged pre-delivery pain in our study. Maternal asthma may increase the risk of adverse fetal and maternal outcomes, such as preterm birth, and, uterine hemorrhage. Therefore, managing pregnant asthmatics requires a careful benefit-risk analysis, and when indicated, the benefits of a medication that may have increased risks can dictate its use in severe uncontrolled asthma [18]. The present research did not identify that asthma worsened as gestation progressed in a linear fashion, with the greater proportion of women experiencing a loss of control rather than an exacerbation. Whereas Luke E. reported that the women who had recurrent bouts of uncontrolled asthma during pregnancy were significantly more likely to have a poor perinatal outcome than the women who had acute exacerbations during pregnancy. This suggests that long periods of uncontrolled asthma may be more harmful than acute exacerbations for the fetus, specifically in relation to fetal growth [4].

Regarding the ethnicity of our study population, Turks had more severe exacerbations than Farsi. Carroll et al. examined ethnic differences in the incidence of asthma exacerbations in a low-income population of pregnant women and noted that the proportion of emergency room presentations and hospital admissions was significantly higher among Blacks than among Whites [3]. This could be due to disparities in access to health care rather than differences in the underlying severity of disease thought. In the present study, only 14.3% of women who were living in village had severe asthma exacerbation, whereas 85.7% women who lived in city had severe asthma exacerbation.

The results of recent studies suggest that factors in rural environments may protect against the development of allergic diseases, but the underlying mechanisms are not well understood. Nonetheless, Lee et al. showed protective factors associated with a farming environment and/or rural lifestyle may influence the prevalence of allergic diseases and atopy in Korean children [19]. We examined potential maternal risk factors for exacerbation, such as age, parity, gravidity, education, smoking; body mass index, asthma control questionnaire (ACQ), and lung function, but found no differences between the women who had a severe exacerbation and those who did not. In line with Murphy et al.'s findings [10], we could not find an association between ACQ and severity of exacerbations. ACQ can be used in the evaluation of asthma control at any point in time [20]. But no such validated tools are available for identifying exacerbations [4]. Therefore, a major strength of this study is that it provides new evidence that an acute exacerbation may be a greater driver for poor perinatal outcomes than chronically or persistently uncontrolled asthma. Other major strength of this study is reflected in the detailed and prospective collection of data on asthma status and perinatal outcomes, although small sample size limited our results.

However, data regarding the association between asthma exacerbations during pregnancy and adverse fetal outcomes are inconclusive due to small sample sizes and the lack of statistical power of numerous studies, the interstudy variations in the characteristics of study populations, the definition of exacerbations and their timing during pregnancy, and the choice of the reference group (women without asthma or asthmatic women without exacerbations) [7].

10. Conclusion

In conclusion, an asthma exacerbation-like allergen exposure during pregnancy was associated with pregnancy complications, including UTI, pain, and bleeding. Prevention of exacerbations is essential to reduce the risk of complications and poor outcome. Novel management strategies must be developed to address the complex needs of pregnant women with asthma. These include medication non-adherence and the presence of numerous comorbidities, which can affect asthma, such as cold symptoms, cigarette smoking, allergy, and mental health issues. Inflammation-based management has been shown to be effective in reducing exacerbations in pregnancy and may also improve perinatal outcomes. The involvement of a multidisciplinary team and the assessment of comorbidities have the potential to improve maternal, fetal, and newborn health, by preventing severe exacerbations.

Appendix

Table 1 compares maternal characteristics between groups, providing insights into demographic and clinical variables. However, most p-values are non-significant, except for "City/Village" (p = 0.03). Significant findings should be emphasized for clarity. Terms like "prehighschool" should be revised to "Pre-High School," and column headers clarified as "No Severe Exacerbation" and "Severe Exacerbation."

Characteristics		No severe exacerbation	Severe exacerbation	P value
Education	Illiterate	2(7.4)	0(0.0)	Fisher's Exact Test = 0.39
	Elementary school	9(33.3)	1(14.3)	
	Pre-high school	7(25.9)	3(42.9)	
	High school	7(25.9)	1(14.3)	
	University education	2(7.4)	2(28.6)	
Age	≤24 years	4(14.8)	1(14.3)	Fisher's Exact Test = 0.07
	25–29 years	6(22.2)	4(57.1)	
	30–34 years	5(18.5)	2(28.6)	
	≥35	12(44.4)	0(0.0)	
Ethnic group	Farsi	13(48.1)	2(28.6)	Fisher's Exact Test = 0.42
	Turk	14(51.9)	5(71.4)	

Characteristics		No severe exacerbation	Severe exacerbation	P value
Gravidity	>2	11(40.7)	4(57.1)	Fisher's Exact Test = 0.67
	<2	16(59.3)	3(42.9)	
Parity	>2	13(48.1)	6(85.7)	Fisher's Exact Test = 0.10
	<2	14(51.9)	1(14.3)	
Smoking	No	25(92.6)	6(85.7)	Fisher's Exact Test = 0.51
	Yes	2(7.4)	1(14.3)	
City/village	City	10(37.0)	6(85.7)	Fisher's Exact Test = 0.03
	Village	17(63.0)	1(14.3)	
Using drug*	Yes	25(92.6)	5(71.4)	
	No	2(7.4)	2(28.6)	Fisher's Exact Test = 0.18
FEV1FVCPRED	Intermittent/mild	25(92.6)	7(100)	Fisher's Exact Test = 1.0
	Persistent moderate	2(7.4)	0(0.0)	
BMI	<19.8	5(18.5)	2(28.6)	Fisher's Exact Test = 0.61
	19.8–26	22(81.5)	5(71.4)	
Fvc* pred	Severe	1(3.7)	0(0.0)	Fisher's Exact Test = 0.64
	Mild	4(14.8)	0(0.0)	
	Intermittent	22(81.5)	7(100)	
Fev*1	Severe	2(7.4)	1(14.3)	Fisher's Exact Test = 0.60
	Mild	4(14.8)	0(0.0)	
	Intermittent	21(77.8)	6(85.7)	
ACQ*	<0.75	8(29.6)	2(28.6)	Fisher's Exact Test = 1.0
	>1.5	12(44.4)	3(42.9)	
	n/a	7(25.9)	2(28.6)	

*Data are presented as Fisher's Exact Test, unless otherwise stated. BMI: body mass index; drug: ICS: inhaled corticosteroid; LABA: long-acting β2-agonist; FEV*1: forced expiratory volume in 1 s; FVC*: forced vital capacity; OCS: oral corticosteroid. ACQ*: asthma control questionnaire.*

Table 1.
Maternal characteristics of women with and without a severe asthma exacerbation during pregnancy.

Table 2 effectively categorizes asthma exacerbation events based on baseline severity. However, some variables, such as "Number wake up at night" (100% across all groups), do not add value and could be summarized. Column labels should be more descriptive, such as "Baseline Intermittent Asthma." Emphasis should be placed on significant differences, such as hospital admission rates.

Table 3 presents laboratory findings, which are critical for understanding physiological differences. Terminology should be standardized, such as "IgE mother" to "Maternal IgE Levels," and units should be added where necessary (e.g., IgE in ng/mL). Significant results or trends should be highlighted to connect laboratory data to clinical outcomes.

Characteristic	Intermittent	Mild asthma	Moderate asthma	Severe asthma	Overall
	N = 13	N = 10	N = 8	N = 3	
Taking regular asthma medicine	6(46.2%)	9(90.0)	3(37.5)	2(66.7)	20(58.8)
Asthma attack three times or more	3(23.1)	2(20.0)	3(37.5)	2(66.7)	10(29.4)
Mother admitted to hospital	3(23.1)	2(20.0)	0(0.0)	0(0.0)	5(14.7)
Number of days when referred to doctor	13(100.0)	10(100.0)	8(100.0)	3(100.0)	34(100.0)
Infant admission	4(30.8)	0(0.0)	0(0.0)	0(0.0)	4(11.8)
Number of days of very poor asthma control	0(0.0)	1(10.0)	0(0.0)	1(33.3)	2(5.9)
Number of times of waking up at night	13(100.0)	10(100.0)	8(100.0)	3(100.0)	34(100.0)
Number of times of using drug in	13(100.0)	10(100.0)	8(100.0)	3(100.0)	34(100.0)
Limitation: low	0(0.0)	1(10)	1(12.5)	2(66.7)	4(11.8)
Moderate	5(38.5)	4(40.0)	3(37.5)	0(0.0)	12(35.3)
Severe	8(61.5)	5(50.0)	4(50.0)	1(33.3)	18(52.9)

Table 2.
Classifications of severe exacerbation events in pregnant women with baseline mild, moderate, or severe asthma.

Characteristic	Intermittent	Mild asthma	Moderate asthma	Severe asthma	Overall
	N = 13	N = 10	N = 8	N = 3	
Maternal IgE level	3(23.1)	3(30.0)	2(25.0)	0(0.0)	8(23.5)
Infant IgE level	13(100.0)	10(100.0)	8(100.0)	3(100.0)	34(100.0)
Eosinophil count mother	12(92.3)	10(100.0)	8(100.0)	3(100.0)	33(97.1)
Eosinophil count infant	12(92.3)	9(90.0)	7(87.5)	1(33.3)	29 (85.3)

Table 3.
Classifications of severe exacerbation events in laboratory in pregnant women with baseline mild, moderate, or severe asthma.

Table 4 provides important data on perinatal outcomes but includes uniform findings (e.g., "Gestational age" is 100% for both groups). Terms like "upper than 2500 mg" should be revised to "Birth weight > 2500 g." Significant outcomes, such as weight gain differences, should be emphasized, and uniform results should be summarized.

Table 5 links allergen exposure to pregnancy complications, emphasizing its clinical relevance. Headings should be clarified, and odds ratios (e.g., OR [95% CI]) formatted consistently. Significant associations, such as "Exposure Allergen and Bleeding" (p = 0.01), should be highlighted. Reorganizing the outcomes into groups (e.g., maternal and fetal outcomes) would improve readability.

Characteristic		No severe exacerbation	Severe exacerbation	P value
Weight gain	0–10 kg	14(51.9)	2(28.6)	Fisher exact test = 0.45
	11–21 kg	11(40.7)	4(57.1)	
	21–30 kg	2(7.4)	1(14.3)	
Birth weight	<2500 mg	1(3.7)	0(0.0)	Fisher's Exact Test = 1
	>2500 mg	26(96.3)	7(100)	
Gestational age	37–42 weeks	27(100)	7(100)	
Blood pressure (BP) high	No	26(96.3)	7(100)	Fisher's Exact Test = 1
	Yes	1(3.7)	0(0.0)	
Vaginal bleeding	No	25(92.6)	7(100)	Fisher's Exact Test = 1
	Yes	2(7.4)	0(0.0)	
Nausea	No	24(88.9)	7(100)	Fisher's Exact Test = 1
	Yes	3(11.1)	0(0.0)	
Method of labor	Vaginal delivery	13(48.1)	3(42.9)	Fisher's Exact Test = 1
	Cesarean	14(51.9)	4(57.1)	
APGAR1	<7	2(7.4)	0(0.0)	Fisher's Exact Test = 1
	>7	25(62.6)	7(100)	
APGAR5	>7	27(100)	7(100)	
Anomaly	No	26(96.3)	7(100.0)	Fisher's Exact Test = 1
	Yes	1(3.7)	0(0.0)	
Gender	Boy	12(44.4)	4(57.1)	Fisher's Exact Test = 0.68
	Girl	15(55.6)	3(42.9)	
Having maternal cold	Yes	19(70.4)	4(57.1)	Fisher's Exact Test = 0.65
	No	8(29.6)	3(42.9)	

Table 4.
Perinatal outcomes in asthmatic women with and without a severe exacerbation during pregnancy.

Characteristic	Possibility	Exposure of allergen	Common cold	Smoke
Bleeding	No	25(96.2%)	32(2.2%)	121(7.5%)
	Yes	7(87.5%)	8(5.6%)	15(10.6%)
P value		0.01	0.48	0.35
OR (95% CI)		0.46(0.29–0.70)	0.46(0.21–2.07)	1.30(0.47–2.30)
Pain 3w before delivery	No	218(14.1%)	39(2.5%)	127(7.5%)
	Yes	14(25.5%)	1(1.8%)	9(16.4%)
P value		0.01	0.76	0.03
OR (95% CI)		0.44(0.23–0.84)	0.68(0.05–8.14)	0.45(0.21–0.95)
PROM 3w before delivery	No	223(14.5%)	40(2.6%)	130(7.7%)
	Yes	9(13.2%)	0(0.0%)	6(8.8%)

Characteristic	Possibility	Exposure of allergen	Common cold	Smoke
P value		0.85	0.99	0.91
OR (95% CI)		1.07(0.50–2.26)	0	0.95(0.40–2.25)
Placenta problem	No	227(14.3%)	38(2.4%)	135(7.8%)
	Yes	5(35.7%)	2(14.3%)	1(7.1%)
P value		0.19	0.47	0.85
OR (95% CI)		0.42(0.11–1.54)	2.57(0.19–34.29)	1.21(0.15–9.41)
Preeclampsia	No	217(14.2%)	39(2.6%)	126(7.5%)
	Yes	15(20%)	1(1.3%)	10(13.3%)
P value		0.17	0.29	0.12
OR (95% CI)		0.65(0.35–1.21)	0.27(0.02–3.04)	0.58(0.29–1.16)
Gestational diabetes	No	227(14.4%)	37(2.4%)	132(7.7%)
	Yes	5(16.7%)	3(10.0%)	4(13.3%)
P value		0.47	0.47	0.34
OR (95% CI)		1.60(0.43–5.93)	2.07(0.29–14.72)	0.59(0.20–1.73)
UTI	No	226(0.15%0	39(2.6%)	126(8.4%)
	Yes	6(6.1%)	1(1.0%)	10(10.2%)
P value		0.04	0.95	0.52
OR (95% CI)		2.32(1.00–5.39)	0.93(0.12–7.14)	080(0.40–1.58)
Vomiting	No	183(14.4%)	30(2.4%)	106(7.4%)
	Yes	49(14.8%)	10(3.0%)	30(9.1%)
P value		0.16	0.38	0.31
OR (95% CI)		1.37(0.87–2.16)	1.60(0.55–4.68)	0.78(0.49–1.25)
Weight of the infant	No	106(7.8%)	124(7.9%)	111(7.6%)
	Yes	20(8.6%)	2(5.0%)	15(11.0%)
P value		0.38	0.98	0.15
OR (95% CI)		1.25(0.75–2.09)	1.02(0.19–5.27)	1.51(0.85–2.68)
Anomaly	No	230(99.1%)	39(97.5%)	134(98.5%)
	Yes	2(0.9%)	1(2.5%)	2(1.5%)
P value		0.85	0.63	0.11
OR (95% CI)		0.n(0.10–6.29)	2.33(0.6–79.77)	0.27(0.55–1.38)

Table 5.
Distribution of various maternal allergen exposures on pregnancy outcomes in two groups.

Author details

Nasrin Fazel[1,2]

1 Iranian Research Center on Healthy Aging, Department of Medical-Surgical Nursing, School of Nursing and Midwifery, Sabzevar University of Medical Sciences, Sabzevar, Iran

2 Department of Environmental Health, Center for Public Health, Medical University Vienna, Vienna, Austria

*Address all correspondence to: shohreh1368@yahoo.co.uk

References

[1] Blais L, Forget A. Asthma exacerbations during the first trimester of pregnancy and the risk of congenital malformations among asthmatic women. Journal of Allergy and Clinical Immunology. 2008;**121**(6):1379-1384 e1

[2] Koo S-M, Kim Y, Park C, Park GW, Lee M, Won S, et al. Effect of pregnancy on quantitative medication use and relation to exacerbations in asthma. BioMed Research International. 20 Jul 2017;**2017**:8276190. DOI: 10.1155/2017/8276190

[3] Yoo EJ, Lee NL, Huang KP, Kose LT, Desai D, Plante LA, et al. Clinical characteristics of severe asthma exacerbations among inner-city women in pregnancy. The Journal of Allergy and Clinical Immunology: In Practice. 2020;**8**(1):395-397

[4] Grzeskowiak LE, Smith B, Roy A, Dekker GA, Clifton VL. Patterns, predictors and outcomes of asthma control and exacerbations during pregnancy: A prospective cohort study. ERJ Open Research. 18 Feb 2016;**2**(1):00054-2015. DOI: 10.1183/23120541.00054-2015. eCollection 2016 Jan

[5] Murphy VE, Clifton VL, Gibson PG. Asthma exacerbations during pregnancy: Incidence and association with adverse pregnancy outcomes. Thorax. 2006;**61**(2):169-176

[6] Firoozi F, Ducharme FM, Lemière C, Beauchesne M-F, Perreault S, Forget A, et al. Effect of fetal gender on maternal asthma exacerbations in pregnant asthmatic women. Respiratory Medicine. 2009;**103**(1):144-151

[7] Blais L, Kettani F-Z, Forget A, Beauchesne M-F, Lemière C. Asthma exacerbations during the first trimester of pregnancy and congenital malformations: Revisiting the association in a large representative cohort. Thorax. 2015;**70**(7):647-652

[8] Ali Z, Ulrik CS. Incidence and risk factors for exacerbations of asthma during pregnancy. Journal of Asthma and Allergy. 2013;**6**:53

[9] Brightling CE. Asthma exacerbations during pregnancy: A need for precision medicine. Respirology. Jul 2020;**25**(7):670-671. DOI: 10.1111/resp.13761. Epub 2019 Dec 16

[10] Murphy VE, Gibson P, Talbot PI, Clifton VL. Severe asthma exacerbations during pregnancy. Obstetrics & Gynecology. 2005;**106**(5):1046-1054

[11] Suzuki K, Shinohara R, Sato M, Otawa S, Yamagata Z. Association between maternal smoking during pregnancy and birth weight: An appropriately adjusted model from the Japan environment and children's study. Journal of Epidemiology. 2016;**26**(7):371-377

[12] Shepardson RL, Hustad JT. Hookah tobacco smoking during the transition to college: Prevalence of other substance use and predictors of initiation. Nicotine & Tobacco Research. 2015;**18**(5):763-769

[13] Schatz M, Dombrowski MP, Wise R, Thom EA, Landon M, Mabie W, et al. Asthma morbidity during pregnancy can be predicted by severity classification. The Journal of Allergy and Clinical Immunology. 2003;**112**:283-288

[14] Asthma Management Handbook. South Melbourne, Australia: National Asthma Council Australia; 2002

[15] Murphy VE, Gibson PG, Giles WB, Zakar T, Smith R, Bisits AM, et al. Maternal asthma is associated with reduced female fetal growth. American Journal of Respiratory and Critical Care Medicine. 2003;**168**:1317-1323

[16] Minerbi-Codish I, Fraser D, Avnun L, Glezerman M, Heimer D. Influence of asthma in pregnancy on labor and the newborn. Respiration. 1998;**65**:130-135

[17] Romero R, Kusanovic JP, Muñoz H, Gomez R, Lamont RF, Yeo L. Allergy-induced preterm labor after the ingestion of shellfish. The Journal of Maternal-Fetal & Neonatal Medicine. 2010;**23**(4):351-359

[18] Rocklin RE. Asthma, asthma medications and their effects on maternal/fetal outcomes during pregnancy. Reproductive Toxicology. 2011;**32**(2):189-197

[19] Lee S, Kwon JW, Seo J, Song Y, Kim B, Yu J, et al. Prevalence of atopy and allergic diseases in Korean children: Associations with a farming environment and rural lifestyle. International Archives of Allergy and Immunology. 2012;**158**(2):168-174

[20] Fazel N, Kundi M, Jensen-Jarolim E, Pali-Schöll I, Kazemzadeh A, Abdi-zadeh MF, et al. Prospective cohort study of pregnancy complications and birth outcomes in women with asthma. Archives of Gynecology and Obstetrics. 2018;**298**(2):279-287

Chapter 7

Asthma-COPD Overlap: Focus on Sex Differences

Yosima Gonzalez and Patricia Silveyra

Abstract

Asthma-COPD Overlap (ACO), also known as asthma-COPD overlap syndrome (ACOS), is a condition where patients exhibit features of both asthma and chronic obstructive pulmonary disease (COPD). Recently, it has been shown that biological sex plays a significant role in ACO. Women with ACO typically experience more severe symptoms, higher rates of exacerbations, and worse quality of life compared to men. Differences in airway anatomy may partly explain this disparity, as women tend to have proportionally smaller airways than men. Additionally, women are often more sensitive to environmental triggers and display stronger inflammatory responses. Hormonal factors such as estrogen levels can also influence airway inflammation and reactivity, contributing to ACO phenotypes. Despite women being more severely affected by ACO, they are often diagnosed later than men, which can lead to delayed treatment and poorer outcomes. In this chapter, we describe the ACO pathophysiology and risk factors, and we discuss the current state of the field in elucidating mechanisms underlying sex differences.

Keywords: asthma, COPD, sex differences, ACOS, lung inflammation, lung disease, women's health

1. Introduction

Asthma-COPD Overlap (ACO), formerly referred to as asthma-COPD overlap syndrome (ACOS), is a clinical phenotype characterized by features of both asthma and chronic obstructive pulmonary disease (COPD) [1]. The term was introduced to acknowledge a subset of patients who defy classical distinctions between these conditions, necessitating a unique clinical approach [2, 3]. Asthma is a chronic respiratory disease characterized by variable airflow obstruction, airway hyperresponsiveness, and inflammation, often with an eosinophilic or allergic background. COPD, in contrast, is defined by persistent, largely irreversible airflow limitation associated with a chronic inflammatory response to inhaled irritants, typically tobacco smoke, air pollution, or biomass fuel exposure. Thus, chronic airway inflammation is a significant factor in ACO and contributes to airway remodeling, airflow obstruction, and multiple disease symptoms, including wheezing and dyspnea, which tend to worsen during acute exacerbations [4].

The public health implications of ACO are substantial, representing a significant population health burden that affects millions of patients with disproportionate impact on socioeconomically disadvantaged populations [5]. The condition serves as a major driver of healthcare costs and resource utilization, highlighting the critical need for targeted screening programs, specialized treatment protocols, and interventions that address the socioeconomic barriers to care that characterize this population [6].

2. Clinical presentation, pathophysiology, and risk factors

Patients with ACO typically present with persistent airflow limitation that shows significant bronchodilator reversibility, along with a history of childhood asthma, allergies, or atopy [7]. These patients typically present at age 40 or older with persistent post-bronchodilator airflow limitation (FEV1/FVC <0.70), characteristic of COPD, combined with significant bronchodilator reversibility (improvement of>15% and > 400 mL in FEV1), typical of asthma [8]. Additional diagnostic criteria include a history of asthma before age 40 or elevated blood eosinophils, at least 10 pack-years of smoking [2, 9], and variable symptoms that often worsen at night or early morning [10].

Since asthma and COPD present with similar symptoms and ACO encompasses multiple phenotypic variations, establishing clear diagnostic criteria has remained challenging [11]. ACO does not result from a single, distinct etiology but rather reflects a convergent pathophysiological process in which risk factors for both asthma and COPD interact along a continuum of airflow obstruction [12]. Thus, the development of ACO typically involves the simultaneous presence of risk factors from both constituent diseases, with cigarette smoking and environmental exposures serving as primary drivers [13].

Tobacco use has emerged as the predominant risk factor for ACO, with epidemiological evidence demonstrating its profound impact on obstructive airway disease development [14]. A large retrospective cohort study revealed that continuous cigarette smoking increased COPD risk nearly five-fold compared to non-smokers (36% versus 8% incidence), establishing smoking as a critical pathway toward ACO development in susceptible individuals [15]. Moreover, among current cigarette smokers, adults with ACO have a notably higher rate of heat tobacco products (HTP) use, with an adjusted odds ratio (OR) of 5.81 compared to smokers without ACO [16]. HTPs are electronic devices designed to heat tobacco leaves, creating aerosols that contain nicotine, carcinogens, additives, and flavored compounds [17].

From a clinical management perspective, ACO presents unique challenges that traditional single-disease approaches often fail to address adequately [18–20]. The complexity of the condition requires the use of combination therapies that target symptoms of both asthma and COPD simultaneously [21], and early identification is crucial to prevent irreversible lung damage [11, 22]. The pathophysiology of ACO involves a complex, dual inflammatory process that combines Type 2 (eosinophilic) inflammation, typical of asthma, with Type 1 (neutrophilic) inflammation characteristic of COPD [13, 23, 24]. This results in a mixed inflammatory profile that contributes to more severe disease than either asthma or COPD alone [25]. Thus, patients with ACO experience more severe symptoms, faster lung function decline, and higher exacerbation rates compared to those with asthma or COPD individually and thus display increased healthcare utilization [26–28]. Effective treatment often requires personalized, combination approaches targeting both asthma and COPD pathways [29, 30].

Another key feature bridging asthma and COPD is airway hyperresponsiveness (AHR) to allergens and environmental triggers. Longitudinal data from 9651 subjects followed for 11 years revealed that heightened AHR independently predicts COPD onset, underscoring this shared pathophysiological pathway in ACO [15]. Furthermore, atopy and early allergic sensitization play essential roles in connecting asthma to subsequent COPD development. An observational study of 1025 men with a mean age of 61 demonstrated that atopic individuals were at significantly higher risk for COPD, suggesting that early allergic inflammation predisposes patients to the mixed inflammatory patterns seen in ACO [4]. Collectively, these findings illustrate how the convergence of smoking-related airway injury, allergic sensitization, and AHR creates a complex pathophysiological environment that leads to ACO development.

3. Epidemiology

The absence of standardized diagnostic criteria for ACO represents a challenge to determining its actual epidemiological burden [31]. Current prevalence estimates suggest that ACO affects approximately 2–3% of the general adult population [5, 8, 32]. When examining ACO within the context of its component diseases, the condition demonstrates considerable prevalence variability, occurring in 2–12% of patients with COPD and 5–17% of those with asthma, depending on the diagnostic criteria and population studied [32, 33]. In some population-based cohorts, approximately 26% of asthma patients and up to 30% of COPD patients meet the criteria for ACO.

In general, ACO is more prevalent among older adults, especially those who have experienced childhood-onset asthma and a significant history of smoking [7]. More recently, multiple studies have reported a higher prevalence of ACO in women, who may also present with more pronounced symptoms and greater health-related quality-of-life impairments [34–37]. However, compared to asthma or COPD alone, ACO is associated with more frequent exacerbations, increased hospitalizations, more extended hospital stays, greater medication use, and higher healthcare resource utilization [11].

Geographic variations in prevalence have also been reported, with estimates ranging from 3.7% in the United States to 0.61% in China, likely reflecting differences in genetic susceptibility, environmental exposures, and diagnostic practices across populations [26, 38, 39]. ACO patients also demonstrate a distinct demographic profile with a mean age of 64.0 years, positioning them younger than typical COPD patients (67.1 years) but older than typical asthma patients (59 years). This age distribution suggests either the occurrence of early-onset COPD with asthmatic features, or progressive asthma that develops fixed obstruction over time [18, 21, 40]. A study in Japan indicated that the incidence could range from 4.2% to 49.7%, depending on the population and criteria used [41]. The same study reported that ACO patients are typically younger than non-ACO COPD patients, have a higher rate of physician-diagnosed asthma, and use more medications, especially inhaled corticosteroids [41].

ACO also presents a substantially greater clinical burden than other obstructive airway diseases [42]. Comorbidity rates are exceptionally high, with an overwhelming 90.2% of ACO patients reporting at least one additional condition. These rates are significantly higher than those of COPD alone (84%) and far exceeding asthma or control populations [5]. Main comorbidities include cardiovascular disease, diabetes, hypertension, depression, anxiety, and metabolic disorders [43, 44]. The high comorbidity burden likely reflects the systemic inflammatory nature of the condition and shared risk factors between respiratory and other chronic diseases. These patients also report higher rates of disability (70.8% compared to 58.6% of those with COPD alone) and work absences, as well as reduced rates of physical activity and lower quality of life scores [5, 45, 46].

The frequent exacerbations and more severe symptom burden translate directly into increased healthcare costs and morbidity, making ACO a major driver of respiratory-related healthcare expenditure [47]. It is estimated that ACO patients experience hospitalization or emergency department visits at a rate nearly double that of those with COPD alone, despite their younger average age, underscoring the severity and complexity of this condition and the urgent need for early identification and targeted management strategies [48].

Finally, notable socioeconomic disparities also characterize the ACO population [6, 49]. These include elevated body mass index (BMI), reduced household income, and diminished educational achievement [50]. These disparities perpetuate a cycle of suboptimal care through diagnostic delays, inadequate specialist access, medication non-adherence, and persistent exposure to disease-exacerbating environmental factors.

4. Sex differences

It has long been recognized that sex-based differences significantly influence the clinical presentation, management, and outcomes of both asthma and COPD [51, 52]. Women with asthma face higher hospitalization and readmission rates than men, despite receiving comparable in-hospital care, and often demonstrating superior baseline lung function and primary care management [53]. For COPD, women tend to be younger at diagnosis, have smoked less, and exhibit better lung function than men, yet they experience more frequent exacerbations, greater dyspnea, and higher morbidity [51, 54, 55]. Imaging studies show that females with COPD have smaller airways and a lower burden of emphysema than males, which, combined with biological and hormonal differences, may contribute to their heightened susceptibility and symptom severity [56, 57]. These anatomical variations, combined with biological and hormonal factors, may explain the increased vulnerability and symptom severity observed in women vs. men with ACO.

Based on the available research, several essential sex differences in ACO exist that parallel and extend beyond the known sex differences in asthma and COPD individually [58, 59]. A study conducted in aboriginal populations showed that ACO represented 1.65 and 3.53% in males and females, respectively, showing that women are more than twice as likely to develop ACO compared to men in this group [60]. Several studies have also suggested that women are at increased risk of ACO compared with men, which aligns with the broader pattern seen in adult asthma, where asthma is more prevalent and more severe in women than men [34, 35, 52, 61, 62].

Tobacco use has also shown a differential impact on the development of lung diseases, including ACO, in men and women [63]. The combination of asthma and tobacco exposure leads to a more rapid decline in lung function, greater symptom burden, increased exacerbations, and a higher prevalence of comorbidities compared to either disease alone [18, 64]. Epidemiological studies have also shown that women with asthma are at high risk of progressing to COPD or ACO as they age, with tobacco use significantly accelerating this transition [18, 35, 65]. A study of more than 10,000 adults in South Carolina found that the prevalence of ACO in women who smoked for >10 years was more than double that of men with a comparable smoking history [34]. In contrast, women and men had a similar prevalence of ACO if they were never smokers. Similarly, in a large cohort of women with asthma, those with a history of cigarette smoking were much more likely to develop ACO, and the risk increased with greater cumulative tobacco exposure and age. Specifically, smoking more than 20 pack-years and being over the age of 60 were the strongest predictors of ACO [64]. This risk is compounded by the observation that women are more susceptible to the harmful pulmonary effects of tobacco than men, likely due to biological differences in airway size, hormonal influences, and metabolic processing of tobacco toxins [66]. Beyond smoking, other individual factors such as lower education, obesity, unemployment, and rural residence have also been shown to contribute to the increased risk of both COPD and ACO in women [2, 67, 68].

Women with ACO not only face a higher risk of disease development but also experience a more rapid decline in lung function, increased symptom burden, and a greater frequency of exacerbations compared to men [15, 69]. They are also particularly vulnerable to environmental exposures such as air pollutants and allergens [70]. Chronic and acute exposures to particulate matter ($PM_{2.5}$ and PM_{10}), nitrogen dioxide (NO_2), ozone (O_3), and other traffic-related pollutants have been linked to accelerated lung function decline, increased symptoms, and heightened exacerbation risk in ACO. Biomass fuel combustion (such as wood, charcoal, and dung) used for cooking or heating is also a significant risk factor for ACO in women in low- and middle-income countries [71]. Exposure to these indoor pollutants has been associated with increased rates of chronic bronchitis, asthma exacerbations, and fixed airflow obstruction [72]. Similarly, repeated exposure to indoor and outdoor allergens, such as dust mites, mold, and pollen, can also contribute to differential ACO development and progression in women and men [73]. Collectively, these exposures may act synergistically with sex-specific genetic and immunological predispositions to accelerate disease progression [13, 74].

The pronounced sex differences observed in ACO likely arise from hormonal mechanisms similar to those driving sex disparities in asthma and COPD individually [52, 75–77]. Female sex hormones, including estrogen and progesterone, exert a significant influence across the lifespan, contributing to poorer asthma control and greater AHR in adult women [77]. These hormonal influences on airway inflammation, bronchial reactivity, and immune modulation are expected to similarly impact the asthmatic component of ACO, potentially contributing to the higher symptom burden and exacerbation rates observed in women.

Research on sex differences in respiratory disease treatment has revealed important patterns that likely apply to ACO management [37, 78]. In asthma, the majority of available literature reports that men respond better than women to both asthma and COPD therapeutics. This suggests that women with ACO having features of both conditions may face particular challenges in achieving optimal treatment responses. This, combined with the sex disparities in ACO prevalence and outcomes, underscores the need for the development of personalized medicine approaches that consider both biological sex differences and gender-related factors in diagnosis, treatment, and management of this complex respiratory condition [37].

5. Disease mechanisms and sex-specific features

Asthma and COPD differ fundamentally in their inflammatory and structural pathologies. Asthma is primarily driven by T-helper 2 (Th2) immune responses, leading to eosinophilic inflammation, elevated levels of pro-inflammatory cytokines (such as interleukins (IL)-4, IL-5, and IL-13), and AHR [13, 52, 75]. In contrast, COPD is primarily characterized by Th1- and Th17-mediated inflammation, marked by neutrophilic infiltration, increased IL-8 and TNFα, oxidative stress, and a protease–antiprotease imbalance, which contributes to tissue destruction and airway remodeling [13, 54]. Consequently, patients with ACO frequently exhibit a mixed inflammatory profile, displaying both eosinophilic and neutrophilic inflammation in bronchoalveolar lavage fluid, sputum, and airway tissues [24, 25]. This hybrid inflammatory pattern likely underlies the severe symptoms and increased exacerbation rates observed in ACO compared with asthma or COPD alone [26, 69].

Biological sex has a significant influence on these inflammatory pathways in both asthma and COPD [54, 60, 79, 80]. Gonadal hormones such as estrogen and progesterone modulate immune responses in women, amplifying Th2 pathways and contributing to heightened eosinophilic inflammation observed in asthma and ACO [13, 52, 75]. Conversely, androgens tend to suppress Th2 inflammation, which may partly explain why prepubertal boys have higher asthma prevalence, while postpubertal women experience greater disease burden [61, 81]. These hormonal effects likely interact with genetic and environmental factors to influence the severity, progression, and unique mixed inflammatory profile of ACO, contributing to the increased symptom burden, more frequent exacerbations, and greater healthcare needs observed in women compared to men.

Preclinical and clinical studies conducted over the past decades have indicated that both genetic and epigenetic factors contribute to the pathogenesis of ACO and related sex differences. Shared susceptibility loci, such as polymorphisms in the ADAM33, ORMDL3, and IL17F genes, have been linked to both asthma and COPD, suggesting a genetic predisposition to overlapping phenotypes [74, 82, 83]. Recent transcriptomic and epigenomic analyses of airway samples have revealed distinct gene expression patterns in ACO patients that overlap with those of asthma and COPD, while also displaying unique molecular profiles [74, 82]. These findings highlight potential targets for precision therapies. For example, differential expression of genes regulating eosinophil function (e.g., IL5RA) and neutrophil chemotaxis (e.g., CXCL8) may influence individual responses to inhaled corticosteroids or biologics targeting Type 2 inflammation [24, 25].

Emerging research has also indicated that sex-specific molecular mechanisms contribute to differences in disease severity and treatment response in ACO. Transcriptomic studies have identified sex-biased gene expression in immune pathways, including those involved in interferon signaling and antigen presentation, suggesting that hormonal regulation of these pathways may exacerbate airway inflammation in women [74, 84]. Additionally, sex-specific epigenetic modifications, such as DNA methylation of genes involved in airway remodeling or oxidative stress responses, may further contribute to differential disease progression [74, 85]. Understanding these complex, intertwined mechanisms is essential for advancing personalized medicine for ACO that integrates sex-specific molecular insights into clinical practice.

6. Conclusion

ACO represents a clinically distinct and epidemiologically significant condition that bridges traditional asthma and COPD categories. The epidemiological evidence demonstrates that this dual diagnosis population, while younger than typical COPD patients, carries a disproportionate burden of comorbidities, disability, and health-care utilization. Clinical recognition and proper management of ACO are essential given the associated healthcare costs, morbidity, and the vulnerable socioeconomic profile of affected patients. The concept remains clinically useful despite evolving terminology, emphasizing the need for individualized care approaches that address both asthmatic and COPD features simultaneously. The substantial population burden and clinical complexity of ACO underscore the importance of continued research, targeted interventions, and specialized care protocols for this challenging patient population.

Conflict of interest

The authors declare that they have no conflicts of interest.

Author details

Yosima Gonzalez and Patricia Silveyra*
Indiana University School of Public Health-Bloomington, Bloomington, IN, USA

*Address all correspondence to: psilveyr@iu.edu

References

[1] Leung C, Sin DD. Asthma-COPD overlap: What are the important questions? Chest. 2022;**161**(2):330-344

[2] Gibson PG, Simpson JL. The overlap syndrome of asthma and COPD: What are its features and how important is it? Thorax. 2009;**64**(8):728-735

[3] Sin DD et al. What is asthma-COPD overlap syndrome? Towards a consensus definition from a round table discussion. The European Respiratory Journal. 2016;**48**(3):664-673

[4] Tu X et al. Asthma-COPD overlap: Current understanding and the utility of experimental models. European Respiratory Review. 2021;**30**(159):190185-190198

[5] Kumbhare S et al. Characteristics and prevalence of asthma/chronic obstructive pulmonary disease overlap in the United States. Annals of the American Thoracic Society. 2016;**13**(6):803-810

[6] Venkata AN. Asthma-COPD overlap: Review of diagnosis and management. Current Opinion in Pulmonary Medicine. 2020;**26**(2):155-161

[7] Fouka E et al. Asthma-COPD overlap syndrome: Recent insights and unanswered questions. Journal of Personalized Medicine. 2022;**12**(5):708-722

[8] Leung JM, Sin DD. Asthma-COPD overlap syndrome: Pathogenesis, clinical features, and therapeutic targets. BMJ. 2017;**358**:j3772

[9] Alsayed AR, Abu-Samak MS, Alkhatib M. Asthma-COPD overlap in clinical practice (ACO_CP 2023): Toward precision medicine. Journal of Personalized Medicine. 2023;**13**(4):677-691

[10] Ding B, Enstone A. Asthma and chronic obstructive pulmonary disease overlap syndrome (ACOS): Structured literature review and physician insights. Expert Review of Respiratory Medicine. 2016;**10**(3):363-371

[11] Hines KL, Peebles RS Jr. Management of the Asthma-COPD overlap syndrome (ACOS): A review of the evidence. Current Allergy and Asthma Reports. 2017;**17**(3):15

[12] Forey BA, Thornton AJ, Lee PN. Systematic review with meta-analysis of the epidemiological evidence relating smoking to COPD, chronic bronchitis and emphysema. BMC Pulmonary Medicine. 2011;**11**:36

[13] Hikichi M, Hashimoto S, Gon Y. Asthma and COPD overlap pathophysiology of ACO. Allergology International. 2018;**67**(2):179-186

[14] Løkke A et al. Developing COPD: A 25 year follow up study of the general population. Thorax. 2006;**61**(11):935-939

[15] de Marco R et al. The coexistence of asthma and chronic obstructive pulmonary disease (COPD): Prevalence and risk factors in young, middle-aged and elderly people from the general population. PLoS One. 2013;**8**(5):e62985

[16] Noguchi S et al. Association of cigarette smoking with increased use of heated tobacco products in middle-aged and older adults with self-reported chronic obstructive pulmonary disease, asthma, and asthma-COPD overlap in Japan, 2022: The JASTIS study. BMC Pulmonary Medicine. 2023;**23**(1):365

[17] Nakama C, Tabuchi T. Use of heated tobacco products by people with chronic diseases: The 2019 JASTIS study. PLoS One. 2021;**16**(11):e0260154

[18] Freiler JF. The asthma-COPD overlap syndrome. Federal Practitioner. 2015;**32**(Suppl. 10):19s-23s

[19] Chang J, Mosenifar Z. Differentiating COPD from asthma in clinical practice. Journal of Intensive Care Medicine. 2007;**22**(5):300-309

[20] Cosentino J et al. Analysis of asthma-chronic obstructive pulmonary disease overlap syndrome defined on the basis of bronchodilator response and degree of emphysema. Annals of the American Thoracic Society. 2016;**13**(9):1483-1489

[21] Bakakos A et al. Asthma with fixed airflow obstruction: From fixed to personalized approach. Journal of Personalized Medicine. 2022;**12**(3):333-347

[22] Albertson TE et al. The pharmacological management of asthma-chronic obstructive pulmonary disease overlap syndrome (ACOS). Expert Opinion on Pharmacotherapy. 2020;**21**(2):213-231

[23] Hardin M et al. The clinical features of the overlap between COPD and asthma. Respiratory Research. 2011;**12**(1):127

[24] Sunata K et al. Inflammatory profile of eosinophils in asthma-COPD overlap and eosinophilic COPD: A multi-omics study. Frontiers in Immunology. 2024;**15**:1445769

[25] Fangal VD et al. Distinct physiological, transcriptomic, and imaging characteristics of asthma-COPD overlap compared to asthma and COPD in smokers. eBioMedicine. 2024;**110**:105453

[26] Vaz Fragoso CA et al. Asthma-COPD overlap syndrome in the US: A prospective population-based analysis of patient-reported outcomes and health care utilization. International Journal of Chronic Obstructive Pulmonary Disease. 2017;**12**:517-527

[27] Chung JW et al. Characteristics and self-rated health of overlap syndrome. International Journal of Chronic Obstructive Pulmonary Disease. 2014;**9**:795-804

[28] Bonten TN et al. Defining asthma–COPD overlap syndrome: A population-based study. European Respiratory Journal. 2017;**49**(5):1602008

[29] Maselli DJ et al. Clinical approach to the therapy of asthma-COPD overlap. Chest. 2019;**155**(1):168-177

[30] Yanagisawa S, Ichinose M. Definition and diagnosis of asthma–COPD overlap (ACO). Allergology International. 2018;**67**(2):172-178

[31] Hosseini M et al. Global prevalence of asthma-COPD overlap (ACO) in the general population: A systematic review and meta-analysis. Respiratory Research. 2019;**20**(1):229

[32] Uchida A, Sakaue K, Inoue H. Epidemiology of asthma-chronic obstructive pulmonary disease overlap (ACO). Allergology International. 2018;**67**(2):165-171

[33] Alshabanat A et al. Asthma and COPD overlap syndrome (ACOS): A systematic review and meta analysis. PLoS One. 2015;**10**(9):e0136065

[34] Wheaton AG et al. Gender and asthma-chronic obstructive pulmonary disease overlap syndrome. The Journal of Asthma. 2016;**53**(7):720-731

[35] To, T et al. Asthma and chronic obstructive pulmonary disease overlap in women. Incidence and risk factors. Annals of the American Thoracic Society. 2018;**15**(11):1304-1310

[36] Sodhi A et al. Sex and gender in lung disease and sleep disorders: A state-of-the-art review. Chest. 2022;**162**(3):647-658

[37] Rogliani P et al. Sex differences in adult asthma and COPD therapy: A systematic review. Respiratory Research. 2022;**23**(1):222

[38] Ding B et al. Asthma-chronic obstructive pulmonary disease overlap syndrome in the urban Chinese population: Prevalence and disease burden using the 2010, 2012, and 2013 China National Health and wellness surveys. International Journal of Chronic Obstructive Pulmonary Disease. 2016;**11**:1139-1150

[39] Song JH et al. Differences in prevalence of asthma-COPD overlap according to different criteria. Medicine (Baltimore). 2018;**97**(36):e12049

[40] Cukic V et al. Asthma and chronic obstructive pulmonary disease (COPD) - Differences and similarities. Materia Socio Medica. 2012;**24**(2):100-105

[41] Hashimoto S et al. Asthma and chronic obstructive pulmonary disease overlap according to the Japanese respiratory society diagnostic criteria: The prospective, observational ACO Japan cohort study. Advances in Therapy. 2021;**38**(2):1168-1184

[42] Pleasants RA et al. Chronic obstructive pulmonary disease and asthma-patient characteristics and health impairment. COPD. 2014;**11**(3):256-266

[43] Akmatov MK et al. Comorbidity profile of patients with concurrent diagnoses of asthma and COPD in Germany. Scientific Reports. 2020;**10**(1):17945

[44] Nielsen M, Bårnes CB, Ulrik CS. Clinical characteristics of the asthma-COPD overlap syndrome--a systematic review. International Journal of Chronic Obstructive Pulmonary Disease. 2015;**10**:1443-1454

[45] Miravitlles M et al. Characterisation of the overlap COPD-asthma phenotype. Focus on physical activity and health status. Respiratory Medicine. 2013;**107**(7):1053-1060

[46] Dierick BJH et al. Work absence in patients with asthma and/or COPD: A population-based study. NPJ Primary Care Respiratory Medicine. 2021;**31**(1):9

[47] Blanchette CM et al. Economic burden in direct costs of concomitant chronic obstructive pulmonary disease and asthma in a Medicare advantage population. Journal of Managed Care Pharmacy. 2008;**14**(2):176-185

[48] Mekov E et al. Update on asthma-COPD overlap (ACO): A narrative review. International Journal of Chronic Obstructive Pulmonary Disease. 2021;**16**:1783-1799

[49] Kim MH et al. Heterogeneity of asthma and COPD overlap. International Journal of Chronic Obstructive Pulmonary Disease. 2018;**13**:1251-1260

[50] Zhu M, Chen A. Epidemiological characteristics of asthma-COPD overlap, its association with all-cause mortality, and the mediating role of depressive symptoms: Evidence from NHANES 2005-2018. BMC Public Health. 2024;**24**(1):1423

[51] Whittaker H et al. Sex differences in asthma and COPD hospital admission, readmission and mortality.

BMJ Open Respiratory Research. 2025;**12**(1):e002808-e002815

[52] Silveyra P, Fuentes N, Rodriguez Bauza DE. Sex and gender differences in lung disease. Advances in Experimental Medicine and Biology. 2021;**1304**:227-258

[53] Zein JG et al. Impact of age and sex on outcomes and hospital cost of acute asthma in the United States, 2011-2012. PLoS One. 2016;**11**(6):e0157301

[54] Czarnota P et al. Sex differences in chronic obstructive pulmonary disease: Implications for pathogenesis, diagnosis, and treatment. International Journal of Molecular Sciences. 2025;**26**(6):2747-2760

[55] Siegfried JM. Sex and gender differences in lung cancer and chronic obstructive lung disease. Endocrinology. 2022;**163**(2):1-8

[56] Milne KM et al. Sex-differences in COPD: From biological mechanisms to therapeutic considerations. Frontiers in Medicine (Lausanne). 2024;**11**:1289259

[57] Hong Y et al. Sex differences of COPD phenotypes in nonsmoking patients. International Journal of Chronic Obstructive Pulmonary Disease. 2016;**11**:1657-1662

[58] Diaz-Guzman E, Khosravi M, Mannino DM. Asthma, chronic obstructive pulmonary disease, and mortality in the U.S. population. COPD. 2011;**8**(6):400-407

[59] Baarnes CB et al. Incidence and long-term outcome of severe asthma-COPD overlap compared to asthma and COPD alone: A 35-year prospective study of 57,053 middle-aged adults. International Journal of Chronic Obstructive Pulmonary Disease. 2017;**12**:571-579

[60] Koleade A et al. Female-specific risk factors associated with risk of ACO (asthma COPD overlap) in aboriginal people. The Journal of Asthma. 2020;**57**(9):925-932

[61] Zein JG, Erzurum SC. Asthma is different in women. Current Allergy and Asthma Reports. 2015;**15**(6):28

[62] Naeem A, Silveyra P. Sex differences in Paediatric and adult asthma. European Medical Journal (EMJ). 2019;**4**(2):27-35

[63] Menson KE, Coleman SRM. Smoking and pulmonary health in women: A narrative review and behavioral health perspective. Preventive Medicine. 2024;**185**:108029

[64] Kiljander T et al. Prevalence of asthma–COPD overlap syndrome among primary care asthmatics with a smoking history: A cross-sectional study. NPJ Primary Care Respiratory Medicine. 2015;**25**(1):15047

[65] James AL et al. Decline in lung function in the Busselton health study: The effects of asthma and cigarette smoking. American Journal of Respiratory and Critical Care Medicine. 2005;**171**(2):109-114

[66] Gan WQ et al. Female smokers beyond the perimenopausal period are at increased risk of chronic obstructive pulmonary disease: A systematic review and meta-analysis. Respiratory Research. 2006;**7**(1):52

[67] Aryal S, Diaz-Guzman E, Mannino DM. Influence of sex on chronic obstructive pulmonary disease risk and treatment outcomes. International Journal of Chronic Obstructive Pulmonary Disease. 2014;**9**:1145-1154

[68] Holtjer JCS et al. Identifying risk factors for COPD and

adult-onset asthma: An umbrella review. European Respiratory Review. 2023;**32**(168):230009-2300026

[69] Menezes AMB et al. Increased risk of exacerbation and hospitalization in subjects with an overlap phenotype: COPD-asthma. Chest. 2014;**145**(2):297-304

[70] Han CH et al. Short-term effects of exposure to particulate matter on hospital admissions for asthma and chronic obstructive pulmonary disease. Medicine (Baltimore). 2022;**101**(35):e30165

[71] Morgan BW et al. Epidemiology and risk factors of asthma-chronic obstructive pulmonary disease overlap in low- and middle-income countries. The Journal of Allergy and Clinical Immunology. 2019;**143**(4):1598-1606

[72] Torres-Duque C et al. Biomass fuels and respiratory diseases: A review of the evidence. Proceedings of the American Thoracic Society. 2008;**5**(5):577-590

[73] Wang B et al. Analysis of allergen positivity rates in relation to gender, age, and cross-reactivity patterns. Scientific Reports. 2024;**14**(1):27840

[74] DeMeo DL. Sex and gender Omic biomarkers in men and women with COPD: Considerations for precision medicine. Chest. 2021;**160**(1):104-113

[75] Shah R, Newcomb DC. Sex bias in asthma prevalence and pathogenesis. Frontiers in Immunology. 2018;**9**:2997

[76] Fuseini H, Newcomb DC. Mechanisms driving gender differences in asthma. Current Allergy and Asthma Reports. 2017;**17**(3):19

[77] Tam A et al. The role of female hormones on lung function in chronic lung diseases. BMC Womens Health. 2011;**11**:24

[78] Jenkins CR et al. Personalized treatment of asthma: The importance of sex and gender differences. The Journal of Allergy and Clinical Immunology. In Practice. 2022;**10**(4):963-971.e3

[79] Sansores RH, Ramírez-Venegas A. COPD in women: Susceptibility or vulnerability? European Respiratory Journal. Jan 2016;**47**(1):19-22

[80] Aryal S, Diaz-Guzman E, Mannino DM. COPD and gender differences: An update. Translational Research. 2013;**162**(4):208-218

[81] Yung JA, Fuseini H, Newcomb DC. Hormones, sex, and asthma. Annals of Allergy, Asthma and Immunology. 2018;**120**(5):488-494

[82] Lopes-Ramos CM et al. Sex-biased regulation of extracellular matrix genes in COPD. American Journal of Respiratory Cell and Molecular Biology. 5 Aug 2024;**72**(1):72-81

[83] Mauvais-Jarvis F et al. Sex and gender: Modifiers of health, disease, and medicine. Lancet. 2020;**396**(10250):565-582

[84] Han MK et al. Female sex and gender in lung/sleep health and disease. Increased understanding of basic biological, pathophysiological, and behavioral mechanisms leading to better health for female patients with lung disease. American Journal of Respiratory and Critical Care Medicine. 2018;**198**(7):850-858

[85] Koo HK et al. Sex-specific associations with DNA methylation in lung tissue demonstrate smoking interactions. Epigenetics. 2021;**16**(6):692-703

Section 5

Differential Diagnosis

Chapter 8

Differential Diagnosis in Childhood Asthma

Mehmet Kılıç and Öner Özdemir

Abstract

Asthma is the most common chronic respiratory disease in childhood. A patient with asthma may experience symptoms such as wheezing, coughing, shortness of breath, and chest tightness. It is worth noting that respiratory symptoms, such as cough, wheezing, and shortness of breath, may also be observed in other acute or chronic diseases, including those unrelated to asthma. For example, persistent bacterial bronchitis (PBB) is one of the most common causes of chronic productive cough in young children (<5 years of age), accounting for approximately 40% of referrals to pediatric pulmonary clinics. PBB should be considered in children whose cough significantly improves within 2 weeks of antibiotic treatment. Suppose a child exhibits atypical symptoms or findings in the history and physical examination that may suggest an alternative diagnosis other than asthma. In that case, further investigations should be conducted for differential diagnosis. Additionally, if a child is not responding to maintenance therapy for asthma, the diagnosis of asthma should first be reconsidered. Since it is known that most children with asthma can be well controlled with basic prophylactic therapy, alternative diagnoses should be considered if a patient continues to complain of severe or recurrent respiratory symptoms despite all basic asthma management strategies.

Keywords: childhood, asthma, diagnosis, differential diagnosis, asthma mimics

1. Introduction

Asthma is the most common chronic respiratory disease in childhood. As a result of studies conducted in different countries, it has been reported that the prevalence of asthma in children around the world varies between 1 and 18%. Children with asthma are often reported to present with symptoms before the age of five. The age of onset of asthma is around 1 year in 30% of cases, and in 80–90% of cases, the first symptoms appear before the age of 4–5 years [1].

2. Differential diagnosis in childhood asthma

The primary objective of this chapter is to review the differential diagnosis of childhood asthma and to provide a clinical overview of all possible asthma mimickers included in the differential diagnosis. To this end, we conducted a systematic literature review of articles published in English about "Differential Diagnosis in Childhood Asthma" through PubMed searches and reviewed various journals. Our search period spanned from 1970 to 2025.

A patient with asthma may experience symptoms such as wheezing, coughing, shortness of breath, and chest tightness. In most patients, more than one of these complaints occurs together. Sometimes, one of these may be the patient's only complaint. However, one point that should not be forgotten during asthma diagnosis is that the statement "not every wheeze and cough is asthma" remains a valid consideration. It is worth noting that respiratory symptoms, such as cough, wheezing, and shortness of breath, may also be observed in other acute or chronic diseases, including those unrelated to asthma. Therefore, it is particularly important to consider and exclude alternative causes that may produce symptoms of wheezing, cough, and shortness of breath before confirming the asthma diagnosis in all age groups during childhood [2–4].

The diagnosis of asthma in childhood is confirmed by the presence of typical clinical findings, a detailed history, physical examination, allergy tests, pulmonary function tests (demonstration of reversibility, variability, or airway hyperresponsiveness), or an objective response to treatment [1]. One of the most important diagnostic methods in evaluating chronic respiratory symptoms in childhood is a detailed history and physical examination. Physicians should be alert for signs and symptoms atypical for asthma in the history and physical examination. To this end, the following are some cautionary tips for alternative diagnoses. In the presence of isolated, persistent, and progressive shortness of breath, non-asthmatic diseases should be at the forefront. Persistent bacterial bronchitis (PBB) should be considered in children whose productive cough decreases significantly within 2 weeks with antibiotic treatment. In addition, the presence of a productive cough should suggest bronchiectasis and chronic suppurative lung diseases. If symptoms start from birth or in the first weeks of life, the child should be investigated for differential diagnosis. The younger the child, the more likely an alternative diagnosis is (e.g., gastroesophageal reflux, cystic fibrosis, aspiration syndrome, immunodeficiency, congenital heart disease, or bronchopulmonary dysplasia). Inspiratory sounds or labored breathing indicate extrathoracic pathological conditions (tracheal or laryngeal disorders). Clubbing, failure to thrive, upper respiratory tract findings, stridor, asymmetric wheezing, nasal polyps, cardiac murmur, neurological developmental delay, central cyanosis, and dextrocardia are important clinical findings that suggest alternative diseases. Patients with feeding problems, vomiting, irritability, hematemesis, and those who do not respond to bronchodilator therapy should be evaluated for gastroesophageal reflux disease (GERD). Sudden onset of respiratory symptoms and/or the presence of concomitant monolateral thoracic sounds strongly supports the suspicion of an endobronchial foreign body. Suppose symptoms occur only during the day (without nighttime cough or wheezing) and begin in the absence of obvious triggers. In that case, asthma cannot be definitively excluded, but other possible diagnoses should be seriously considered [1, 3, 5]. If any of the following symptoms or signs are present in children with recurrent respiratory complaints, a diagnosis of asthma is generally ruled out, and further investigations for an alternative diagnosis are warranted (**Tables 1** and **2**).

Spirometric tests, which measure forced expiratory flow in the diagnosis of asthma, can be performed on children over five years of age who are able to cooperate. In recent years, new devices have been used to measure lung function in young children. Unlike forced expiratory maneuvers, these measurements are performed

- Symptoms begin in the neonatal period
- Isolated cough without other respiratory symptoms (except cough variant asthma)
- If symptoms only occur during the day
- Presence of chronic sputum production (cough seen in asthmatic patients is often dry, with small amounts of sticky sputum)
- Accompanied by purulent sputum
- Presence of chest pain, hemoptysis
- Wheezing increases or decreases with a position change
- Accompanied by chronic diarrhea, steatorrhea, failure to thrive
- Respiratory symptoms accompanied by vomiting
- Increased wheezing, respiratory distress, and cough during or after feeding
- Persistent wheezing, rhonchi, and rales
- Recurrent stridor or barking cough
- Symptoms are not associated with typical triggers such as viral upper respiratory tract infections
- If symptoms appear suddenly without a clear triggering factor
- Presence of focal lung findings or clubbing
- Detection of nasal polyps with respiratory symptoms
- Presence of murmur, cyanosis, significant anemia, dextrocardia, and situs inversus with respiratory symptoms
- Presence of hypoxia other than infections and attacks
- Presence of wheezing, rhonchi, and rales that do not respond to asthma treatment

Table 1.
Clinical clues for the differential diagnosis of non-asthma in children with respiratory symptoms [1, 3].

Clinical clue	Possible diagnosis
Perinatal and family history	
Symptoms present from birth	Chronic lung disease in premature infants, PCD, CF
Family history of unusual chest disease	CF, Neuromuscular disorders, PCD
Severe upper respiratory tract disease	PCD
Symptoms and signs	
Persistent moist cough	PBB, bronchiectasis, recurrent aspiration, PCD, CF
Excessive vomiting	Gastroesophageal reflux disease (with/without aspiration)
Dysphagia	Swallowing problems (with/without aspiration)
Breathlessness with lightheadedness and peripheral tingling	Dysfunctional breathing, panic attacks
Inspiratory stridor	Tracheal or laryngeal disorder
Abnormal voice or cry	Laryngeal problems
Persistent wheeze	Extrinsic intrathoracic airway compression, Airway malacia, luminal obstruction, CF, FB
Finger clubbing	CF, bronchiectasis
Failure to thrive	CF, GERD

Abbreviations: CF: Cystic fibrosis; FB: Foreign body; GERD: Gastroesophageal reflux disease; PBB: Protracted bacterial bronchitis; PCD: Primary ciliary dyskinesia.

Table 2.
Alternative diagnoses should be considered based on clinical clues in children with wheezing [3].

during inhalation and exhalation at tidal volumes. In this context, impulse oscillometry (IOS) testing, which does not require patient cooperation, can be used to assess respiratory functions in children under five years of age. This test evaluates lung function by measuring the reflection of sound waves sent from the device in the airways and determining the resistance and reactance values of the airway. This technique appears to be advantageous compared to other respiratory function testing methods because it is effective in evaluating all respiratory tracts in children and requires minimal patient compliance. However, there are difficulties in evaluating the results due to the lack of a sufficient number of studies and the lack of clarity regarding normal values by age group [6].

Additionally, lung function tests can be performed on infants using infant lung function test (iPFT) devices. However, these devices are not available in many centers. Possible interventions in this age group include the tidal breathing flow-volume loop maneuver, rapid thoracoabdominal compression, elevated the raised volume rapid thoracoabdominal compression maneuvers, and lung volume measurement using body plethysmography. In infant lung function testing, tidal volume, respiratory rate, time to peak expiratory flow (as a percentage of total expiratory time), and the pattern of flow/volume loops are usually reported [7].

Fractional exhaled nitric oxide (FeNO) measurement can also be used as an adjunctive test to aid in the diagnosis of asthma. When combined with spirometric measurement and airway hyperresponsiveness, the specificity and sensitivity of FeNO for diagnosing asthma were reported to be 94 and 93%, respectively. FeNO is elevated in asthma, characterized by type 2 inflammation, and can be measured in children over five years of age. In addition to asthma, FeNO may also increase in conditions such as eosinophilic bronchitis, allergic rhinitis, and eczema. Elevation of FeNO is not observed in neutrophilic asthma. FeNO can be used to differentiate nonallergic diseases, such as GERD, vocal cord dysfunction, primary ciliary dyskinesia, and cystic fibrosis, which can be confused with asthma [8]. Finally, in older children, if clinical features suggest asthma but spirometric tests are normal, bronchial challenge testing and exercise challenge testing can be performed. A negative bronchoprovocation test reduces the likelihood of a child having asthma [1]. The asthma diagnostic algorithm for children and adolescents aged 5–16 is given in **Figure 1** [9].

In preschool children, going from treatment to diagnosis is a method used in the diagnosis of asthma. In these children, if the history, physical examination, and laboratory test results do not suggest an alternative diagnosis, but the suspicion of asthma is high, a therapeutic trial with inhaled corticosteroids (average duration of 4–6 weeks) may be considered. However, in older children, documentation of variable airway obstruction is recommended before making a diagnosis of asthma to avoid overdiagnosis and overtreatment. In children with suspected asthma, there are three options for the doctor after treatment is used for diagnostic purposes. First, if there is a response to asthma control treatment, the treatment should be stopped to ensure that the child is not recovering by chance. The same treatment can be started again when symptoms recur. In preschool children, symptom improvement with control treatment is one of the most important clues supporting an asthma diagnosis. Second, if symptoms partially improve despite appropriate treatment, comorbid diseases such as gastroesophageal reflux, dysfunctional breathing, obstructive sleep apnea, and rhinosinusitis accompanying asthma may be considered. The patient should be re-evaluated, and if necessary, treatment should be supplemented to consider these comorbid diseases. Third, if a child is not responding to maintenance therapy for asthma, the diagnosis of asthma should first be reconsidered. Later,

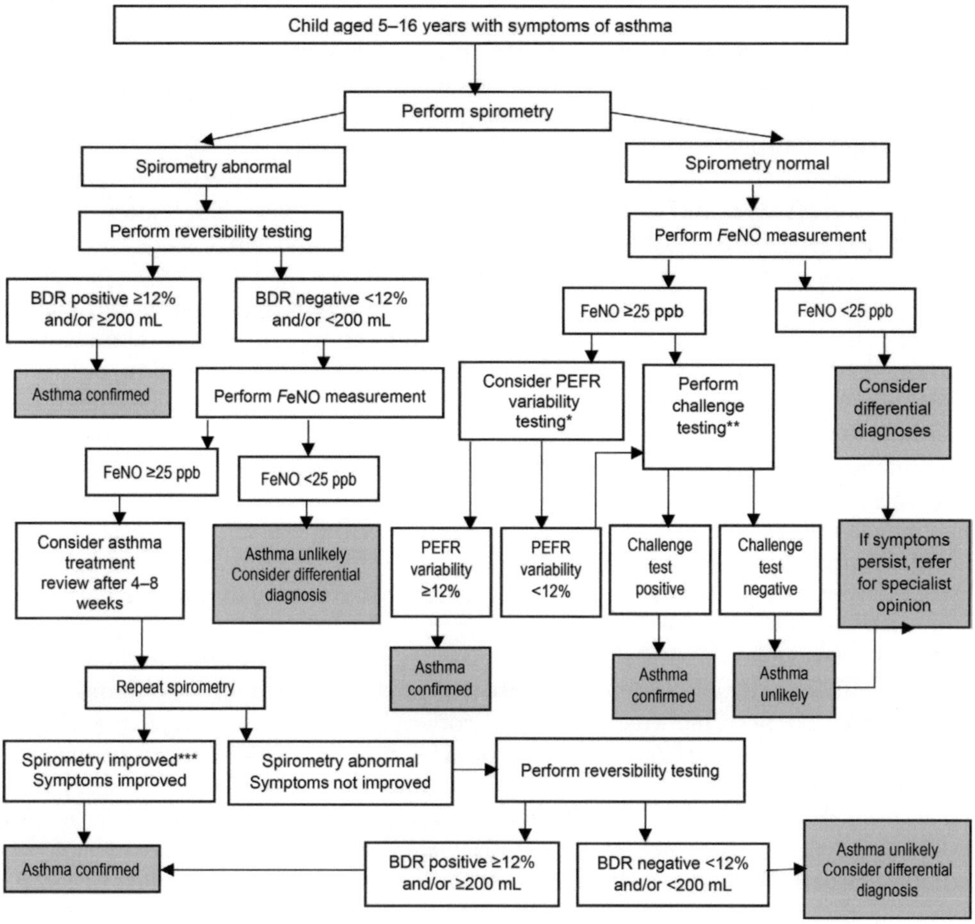

Figure 1.
*An asthma diagnostic algorithm for children and young people aged 5–16 years [9]. Abbreviations: BDR: Bronchodilator reversibility, FeNO: Exhaled nitric oxide fraction, PEFR: Peak expiratory flow rate. *It can be used instead of provocation testing in healthcare facilities where provocation testing is not possible, but this will be an inferior option. **Direct bronchial challenge testing with methacholine or indirect bronchial challenge testing using a treadmill, bicycle, or both can be performed. *** An improvement in FEV1 of more than 7% is considered significant.*

noncompliance with medications or inadequate inhalation technique, persistent environmental exposures, comorbidities (GERD, rhinosinusitis, dysfunctional breathing and/or vocal cord dysfunction, obstructive sleep apnea, and obesity), and psychosocial factors should be questioned. If the child is not diagnosed with asthma as a result of this evaluation, asthma treatment should be discontinued. Because if there is no response to asthma control treatment, the diagnosis of asthma is very unlikely. Subsequently, the patient should be investigated for atypical symptoms or findings that may indicate an alternative diagnosis, and laboratory tests should be performed. For this purpose, the following tests may be ordered for the differential diagnosis of asthma; sweat test and genetic testing for cystic fibrosis; electron microscopy, echocardiography, abdominal ultrasound, and genetic testing for primary ciliary dyskinesia; quantitative immune globulins and lymphocyte panel for immunodeficiencies; chest CT scan for bronchiectasis and bronchiolitis obliterans; sputum or bronchoalveolar lavage culture for persistent bacterial bronchitis; telecardiography, electrocardiography, echocardiography, and cardiac magnetic resonance imaging for congenital heart disease; alpha-1 antitrypsin level and genetic testing for alpha-1 antitrypsin deficiency; chest X-ray and bronchoscopy for foreign body aspirations; pH monitoring, endoscopy, and reflux scintigraphy for gastroesophageal reflux; and fluoroscopy and bronchoscopy for tracheobronchomalacia [2, 3, 5, 10].

The differential diagnosis of childhood asthma can be classified into three groups: Children under five years of age, school-age children, and adolescents. Anatomical and physiological characteristics differ between children under five years of age and those over five years of age. Therefore, clinical findings, diagnosis, and differential diagnosis methods of asthma in children under five years of age present some differences. It is difficult to make a definitive diagnosis of asthma in children five years of age and younger. It is not possible to functionally assess airway obstruction, airflow limitation, or bronchodilator response because of the difficulty of patient compliance. The diagnosis of asthma in young children is largely based on clinical findings [11, 12]. When evaluating infants under 12 months of age for wheezing, the younger the child, the more likely they are to have an alternative diagnosis rather than asthma. The first episode of wheezing before 12 months of age is usually due to bronchiolitis rather than asthma. The differential diagnosis of asthma in children under five years of age should primarily include genetic diseases such as cystic fibrosis, primary ciliary dyskinesia, and immunodeficiency, congenital respiratory and circulatory system anomalies, recurrent viral respiratory infections, foreign body aspiration, persistent bacterial bronchitis, bronchopulmonary dysplasia, and exposure to cigarette smoke. Viral respiratory tract infection has been reported as the most common cause of wheezing in preschool children. In the differential diagnosis of asthma in school-aged children, recurrent respiratory tract infections, chronic upper respiratory tract cough syndrome, bronchiectasis, bronchiolitis obliterans, GERD, tuberculosis, and persistent bacterial bronchitis should be considered first. Adolescence is associated with some differences in terms of asthma. The main differences are smoking habits, obesity, GERD, and failure to comply with long-term treatment during this period. In the differential diagnosis of asthma in adolescence, the following conditions should be considered first: GERD, bronchiectasis, tuberculosis, chronic upper respiratory tract cough syndrome, vocal cord dysfunction, smoking, psychogenic cough, alpha-1 antitrypsin deficiency, hyperventilation, and dysfunctional breathing [1, 3, 9]. **Table 3** lists their typical features of the diseases that should be considered in the differential diagnosis of childhood asthma.

2.1 Respiratory tract infections

The first years of life are the period when children become acquainted with viral and bacterial infections. Therefore, viral lower respiratory tract infections play a significant role among the causes of recurrent wheezing. Recurrent wheezing is common in children under 5 years of age, and the most common cause is viral respiratory infections. Rhinovirus, followed by RSV infections, is the most common cause of wheezing in all age groups [13]. Approximately half of children develop their first episode of wheezing with acute viral bronchiolitis during their first year of life. Approximately 40% of these patients experience recurring wheezing attacks in later years. Therefore, it is essential to remember that a preschool child who experiences one or more episodes of wheezing or dry cough associated with a cold or upper respiratory tract infection early in life should not be diagnosed with asthma. Many of these patients are actually "healthy" children who will not develop wheezing and respiratory symptoms at school age. However, it should not be forgotten that asthma typically begins in early

Diseases	Typical features
Recurrent respiratory tract infections	Mostly cough, runny and stuffy nose lasting <10 days, wheezing usually mild, no symptoms between infections
Upper airway cough syndrome	Sneezing, itching, nasal congestion, throat clearing
Gastroesophageal reflux	Cough during feeding, recurrent lung infections, vomiting after meals, especially large particles, poor response to asthma medications, good response to proton pump inhibitor therapy
Tracheoesophageal fistula and laryngeal cleft	Complaints of wheezing, coughing, and cyanosis occur after feeding
Foreign body aspiration	During feeding or playing, sudden, severe cough and/or stridor, choking attack Recurrent lung infections and cough, focal lung findings, unilateral monophonic wheezing, focal hyperinflation of the lung
Protracted bacterial bronchitis	Persistent wet cough, lung crackles, poor response to asthma medications, good response to long-term antibiotic therapy
Respiratory tract malacia	Persistent stridor/wheezing from birth and severe cough, inspiratory or expiratory retraction may be seen. Symptoms are especially worse when crying or eating, and infections may worsen additional symptoms Poor response to asthma medications
Laryngeal web Tracheal stenosis	Persistent stridor/wheezing from birth; symptoms may increase with infections
Vascular ring	Stridor/wheezing from birth that can change with position Poor response to asthma medications
Congenital anomalies of the lung*	Recurrent or persistent wheezing and coughing since birth
Pulmonary sequestration	Recurrent or persistent wheezing and coughing since birth Decreased breath sounds in a specific area
Tuberculosis	Persistent noisy breathing and cough, fever unresponsive to usual antibiotics, lymphadenopathy, poor response to bronchodilators or inhaled corticosteroids. History of contact with someone with tuberculosis
Congenital heart disease	Cardiac murmur, cyanosis on feeding, fatigue, failure to thrive, tachycardia, tachypnea, or hepatomegaly, poor response to asthma medications
Cystic fibrosis	Symptoms begin shortly after birth and are characterized by recurrent chest infections, a productive cough, failure to thrive, malabsorption, steatorrhea, and bacterial colonization of the airways
Non-cystic fibrosis bronchiectasis	Recurrent infections, productive cough
Primary ciliary dyskinesia	Respiratory distress in newborn babies, persistent rhinitis, sinusitis, otitis, and bronchiolitis from birth Wet cough and recurrent lung infections Persistent purulent/nonpurulent nasal discharge from birth, 50% situs inversus, poor response to asthma medications
Alpha-1 antitrypsin deficiency	Cough with phlegm, wheezing, shortness of breath, family history of early emphysema, liver disease
Vocal cord dysfunction	Dyspnea, expiratory stridor, no reversibility in pulmonary function test No structural abnormalities, no response to asthma medications
Bronchopulmonary dysplasia	Premature and very low birth weight infants requiring prolonged mechanical ventilation or supplemental oxygen Difficulty breathing since birth
Bronchiolitis obliterans	History of severe viral respiratory tract infection in the first 3 years of life Persistent and progressive wheezing, cough, tachypnea, and hypoxia following a severe respiratory tract infection

Diseases	Typical features
Immunodeficiency	Recurrent fever and infections (including non-respiratory), failure to thrive
Psychogenic/habitual cough	Long-term dry, hoarse cough, complaints increase in crowded environments, no cough during sleep No physical findings
Hyperventilation, dysfunctional breathing	Dizziness, paresthesia, sighing

*Abbreviations: *Cystic adenomatoid malformation, bronchial/lung cyst, congenital lobar emphysema, aberrant tracheal bronchus, bronchial stenosis.*

Table 3.
Differential diagnosis of childhood asthma [1, 3].

childhood, and the first symptom of an asthmatic child is usually wheezing, which occurs with viral infections. For this reason, determining whether recurrent wheezing triggered by a virus is asthma has been a research topic in the scientific world for many years [14, 15]. In recurrent respiratory tract infections, symptoms such as cough, nasal congestion, and wheezing typically last less than 10 days. There is no wheezing during periods when there is no infection. It is distinguished from asthma in that the complaints are not recurrent and do not last long [16].

2.2 Foreign body aspiration

Foreign body aspiration in the respiratory tract can occur at any age. However, it is more common in children under four years of age (most commonly between 8 months and 4 years of age). If there are sudden-onset respiratory symptoms, foreign body aspiration should be considered before asthma in this age group. Usually, the patient's history includes the sudden onset of cough, choking, retching, wheezing, cyanosis, and respiratory distress. However, the absence of such a history does not necessarily exclude the diagnosis. The most common clinical findings are persistent cough, unilateral and monophonic wheezing, decreased breath sounds, and respiratory distress [3, 17]. For this reason, some patients may be mistakenly diagnosed and treated for asthma. In patients who do not respond well to asthma treatment and have persistent respiratory symptoms, foreign body aspiration should be considered, and the history should be re-examined from this perspective. Bronchoscopy should be considered, especially in children with localized auscultatory findings and focal radiological findings that may be related to a foreign body [3].

2.3 Protracted bacterial bronchitis

Protracted bacterial bronchitis (PBB) is one of the important causes of chronic cough in childhood. Children with PBB are mostly younger than 5 years old, and despite a prolonged productive cough, their general condition is good, with no growth or developmental delay. In these patients, there is no evidence of sinusitis or otitis, and lung function tests are usually normal [18–20]. The most common microorganisms detected in bronchoalveolar lavage materials taken from patients are *Haemophilus influenzae*, *Streptococcus pneumoniae*, and *Moraxella catarrhalis*. PBB should be considered in children who have a productive cough for more than 4 weeks and whose cough improves significantly within 2 weeks of antibiotic treatment. PBB is often misdiagnosed as asthma, resulting in inappropriate and often high doses of inhaled corticosteroids. Patients with PBB are distinguished from those with asthma by their lack of response to bronchodilator therapy and the presence of expiratory rhonchi and rales, rather than wheezing, on auscultation. However, it should not be forgotten that asthma and PBB can occur together [3]. In untreated cases, PBB carries the risk of causing chronic suppurative lung disease and bronchiectasis [20].

2.4 Cystic fibrosis

The younger the age of onset of cough and wheezing, the higher the probability of congenital malformation, cystic fibrosis, or primary ciliary dyskinesia. The most common findings in children with cystic fibrosis (CF) or non-CF bronchiectasis included in the differential diagnosis of asthma are persistent cough and sputum production. Prolonged sputum production is not a typical finding for asthma, and CF or non-CF bronchiectasis should be considered in these children [21]. Additionally, steatorrhea, growth retardation, nasal polyposis, and pansinusitis may also occur in cystic fibrosis patients. Cystic fibrosis must be excluded in a child with nasal polyps. Although cystic fibrosis is in the newborn screening program, some patients remain undiagnosed due to false-negative results. These patients may present with symptoms such as recurrent cough and wheezing in the early stages of life and be mistakenly diagnosed with asthma [21]. On the other hand, it should not be forgotten that cystic fibrosis and asthma may coexist in a patient [22]. Sweat chloride testing is the first and most important test in diagnosing CF. Genetic testing is used to confirm the diagnosis or to evaluate patients with intermediate sweat test results. If a definitive diagnosis cannot be made with clinical symptoms, sweat test, and molecular methods, in selected patients, additional tests such as nasal potential difference and intestinal flow measurement may be useful [21].

2.5 Non-cystic fibrosis bronchiectasis

Non-cystic fibrosis bronchiectasis remains an important cause of morbidity and mortality in developing countries. The most common findings in children with non-cystic fibrosis bronchiectasis are productive cough, especially in the morning, respiratory distress, and night sweats. The underlying cause can only be determined in 40–63% of these patients. Studies support the etiology of past infections in 69% of cases [23, 24]. On physical examination, auscultatory findings suggestive of airway damage and increased secretion (secretory rales) or clubbing of the fingers are indicative of bronchiectasis. Bronchial dilatation, volume loss, bronchial wall thickening, compensatory hyperinflation, and cyst formation may be seen on chest radiography. The most commonly used test to confirm the diagnosis of bronchiectasis is high-resolution computed tomography [24].

2.6 Primary ciliary dyskinesia

Primary ciliary dyskinesia (PCD) is a genetic disease resulting from a defect in the structure or function of cilia. Unexplained respiratory distress in the newborn baby, persistent rhinitis from birth, sinusitis, otitis, bronchiolitis, pneumonia, bronchiectasis, clubbing of fingers, and situs inversus in 50% of cases are typical findings for primary ciliary dyskinesia. Persistent purulent/nonpurulent rhinitis starting from birth may be a clue for primary ciliary dyskinesia [3]. These children suffer from chronic moist cough, often triggered by viral infections, and are therefore often misdiagnosed as having asthma. Nasal nitric oxide (nNO) measurement is a useful screening tool for diagnosing PCD. Nasal NO levels are extremely low in PCD compared to healthy controls. The gold standard diagnostic method for PCD is the examination of a cilia biopsy taken from the nose or lower respiratory tract. However, when these diagnostic tests are not sufficient in some patients, diagnosis should be supported by genetic analysis [25].

2.7 Alpha-1 antitrypsin deficiency

Alpha-1 antitrypsin (AAT) deficiency is a genetic disease that can cause major lung and liver damage. Some patients with AAT deficiency may be asymptomatic. In symptomatic patients, symptoms usually appear between the ages of 20 and 50. The most common disease caused by AAT deficiency is early-onset panacinar emphysema. Lung symptoms usually include chronic productive cough, shortness of breath, and wheezing. The incidence of bronchiectasis in AAT deficiency has been reported to be 26–43% in various studies [26].

2.8 Bronchiolitis obliterans

Bronchiolitis obliterans (BO) is characterized by persistent and progressive symptoms that occur secondary to infections (e.g., influenza, parainfluenza, measles, respiratory syncytial virus, varicella, and Mycoplasma pneumoniae), most commonly adenovirus. Patients present with persistent wheezing, dyspnea, tachypnea, and cough that are unresponsive to short-acting beta-2 agonists. In these patients, a mosaic perfusion pattern on lung tomography is a characteristic finding [27].

2.9 Bronchopulmonary dysplasia

Bronchopulmonary dysplasia (BPD) is a chronic lung disease that typically occurs in premature and very low birth weight infants as a result of barotrauma and oxygen toxicity caused by mechanical ventilation in early life. BPD should often be considered as the cause of wheezing in children with a history of long-term mechanical ventilation and oxygen support. Patients may complain of visual disturbances, tachypnea, retraction, apnea, cyanosis, and respiratory distress. Rales are often audible during a physical examination. BPD can also cause growth retardation [28].

2.10 Airway malacia

Airway malacia (also known as bronchomalacia, laryngomalacia, or tracheomalacia) is the most common congenital airway anomaly in children. Wheezing heard during expiration indicates an obstruction in the distal airways, while wheezing heard during inspiration should suggest extrathoracic obstruction, and biphasic wheezing should suggest an obstruction in the large central airways. In a child, wheezing, most pronounced during inspiration, indicates congenital laryngeal or tracheal narrowing. The cartilage in the airways is softer than normal, causing lung collapse and respiratory symptoms [29]. In addition, acquired tracheomalacia occurs in the trachea that has been damaged by external pressure (such as tumors, cysts, goiter, or vascular structures), trauma (including tracheostomy), positive-pressure ventilation, infection, or inflammation [30]. In infants, wheezing that can be heard without a stethoscope is usually a sign of a congenital airway lesion. Additionally, laryngomalacia may be suspected when positional stridor occurs in infants. Usually, respiratory complaints (monophonic wheezing and stridor) occur when the child is active (feeding, crying). Advanced airway malacia may lead to apnea, cyanosis, and even the need for respiratory support [30].

2.11 Congenital anomalies

Wheezing that begins soon after birth is probably the result of a congenital anatomical anomaly. Feeding history can provide us with important information about wheezing in childhood. Vomiting and coughing after eating in a wheezy child suggests gastroesophageal reflux disease. However, in rare cases of isolated tracheo-esophageal fistulas and laryngeal clefts, choking, coughing, wheezing, and bruising may occur during feeding. In children with wheezing that occurs with position changes, vascular rings, and major vessel anomalies, as well as tracheomalacia and laryngomalacia, these conditions should be considered [31].

2.12 Gastroesophageal reflux disease

When respiratory problems are accompanied by significant gastroesophageal symptoms, including GERD, recurrent aspiration, and swallowing problems, these conditions should be investigated. GERD can cause respiratory symptoms due to microaspiration, acid stimulation of the esophagus, and stimulation of the vagus nerve. GERD can be a cause of recurrent cough and wheezing, especially in early childhood. In young children, symptoms, such as loss of appetite, vomiting, restlessness, atypical crying, sleep disorders, apnea, and wheezing, are more evident. In later stages, growth retardation may also be observed in children with GERD due to nutritional deficiencies. Wheezing after feeding, frequent vomiting, prominent nocturnal symptoms, and lack of response to bronchodilator therapy are specific to GERD. In adolescents, typical symptoms include a burning sensation in the chest, vomiting, belching, and a bitter taste in the mouth. GERD can also trigger vocal cord dysfunction, which can lead to laryngeal dysfunction and mimic asthma symptoms. Furthermore, GERD symptoms often coexist in children with severe asthma [32, 33]. In symptomatic children, evaluation of response to proton pump inhibitor therapy is recommended as the initial diagnostic method [33].

2.13 Cigarette smoke exposure

Cigarette smoke exposure is an important risk factor for wheezing in children. Maternal smoking during pregnancy and the postnatal period has been found to cause wheezing in the first year and to be associated with lower lung function thereafter. It should be kept in mind that exposure to passive cigarette smoke may also be a factor in children with wheezing whose cause cannot be determined [34].

2.14 Tuberculosis

In patients with persistent, noisy cough, fever, night sweats, weight loss, and a poor response to inhaled corticosteroid treatment without reversibility, tuberculosis contact should be questioned, and tuberculosis should be investigated [35].

2.15 Congenital heart diseases

In children with recurrent respiratory symptoms, cardiac murmur, cyanosis, tachycardia, tachypnea, chest pain, and developmental delay, congenital heart disease should be suspected, and further examinations should be performed. Sometimes asthmatic patients may present with chest pain alone, without cough or wheezing. These patients are defined as chest pain variant asthma. The reversibility test in respiratory function tests may guide the diagnosis of these patients [36].

2.16 Psychogenic/habitual cough

In patients with a noisy, popping cough and no complaints at night, the possibility of a behavioral cough should be considered. Habitual cough is usually seen in crowded environments and during daylight hours. Often, these children come to the doctor's visit with a severe cough and have used numerous treatments, including asthma medications, without benefit. A cough usually begins following an upper respiratory tract infection and can sometimes last for weeks. It is more common in children over eight years of age and can cause extreme distress for both children and parents. The cough disappears at night during sleep or when the child is distracted. The cause of the cough is often unclear, although some children may have mild asthma. Diagnosis is made after other potential causes of cough have been ruled out. Factors that may cause psychological stress in the child's school and home life should be investigated. Some patients respond well to breathing exercises given by a psychotherapist [3].

2.17 Vocal cord dysfunction

As a result of inappropriate movements of the vocal cords (adduction movement during inspiration), inspiratory airflow decreases, leading to intermittent inspiratory symptoms. These patients typically present with complaints such as sudden onset and short-term wheezing, stridor, chest tightness, voice changes, air hunger, shortness of breath triggered by exercise or psychosocial stress, local irritation, or reflux. Initially, the symptoms of vocal cord dysfunction (VCD) were thought to mimic asthma, but recent studies support the notion that VCD is often associated with asthma [37]. Studies are showing that VCD accompanies 35% of patients with severe asthma and 20% of patients with mild asthma. History is important in diagnosis. Spirometry shows findings suggestive of variable extrathoracic obstruction. The gold standard for diagnosis is the visualization of paradoxical movements of the vocal cords during inspiration and expiration with a flexible fiberoptic laryngoscope during an acute attack [37, 38].

2.18 Immunodeficiency

Chronic sinusitis, otitis media, or lower respiratory tract infections (such as pneumonia, bronchitis, bronchiectasis, and interstitial lung diseases) can be frequently observed in patients with immune deficiency. Malabsorption and failure to thrive delay development in some patients [39].

In conclusion, it is well established that most children with asthma can be effectively controlled with basic prophylactic treatment. Therefore, if a child continues to complain of severe or recurrent respiratory symptoms despite all basic asthma management strategies, an alternative diagnosis should be considered. Additionally, children should be evaluated for diseases that mimic asthma if atypical findings for asthma are present in the medical history and physical examination.

Summary box. If any of the following findings are present along with respiratory symptoms, the diagnosis of asthma may be ruled out.

- Onset of symptoms from the neonatal period
- Purulent sputum and hemoptysis accompany the symptoms
- Presence of focal lung findings, cardiac murmur, situs inversus, and clubbing
- Chronic diarrhea, steatorrhea, growth failure, and failure to thrive accompany the respiratory symptoms
- Presence of persistent wheezing, rhonchi, and rales that do not respond to asthma treatment

Author details

Mehmet Kılıç[1*] and Öner Özdemir[2]

1 Department of Pediatric Allergy and Immunology, Fırat University Faculty of Medicine, Elazığ, Turkey

2 Department of Pediatric Allergy and Immunology, Sakarya University Faculty of Medicine, Sakarya, Turkey

*Address all correspondence to: drmkilic@gmail.com

References

[1] Global Initiative for Asthma. Global Strategy for Asthma Management and Prevention. 2025. Available from: www.ginasthma.org

[2] Bergamini M, Kantar A, Cutrera R, Interest Group IPC. Analysis of the literature on chronic cough in children. Open Respiratory Medicine Journal. 2017;**11**:1-9. DOI: 10.2174/1874306401711010001

[3] Ullmann N, Mirra V, Di Marco A, Pavone M, Porcaro F, Negro V, et al. Asthma: Differential diagnosis and comorbidities. Frontiers in Pediatrics. 2018;**6**:276. DOI: 10.3389/fped.2018.00276

[4] Doherty G, Bush A. Diagnosing respiratory problems in young children. The Practitioner. 2007;**251**(20):22-25

[5] Bush A, Grigg J, Saglani S. Managing wheeze in preschool children. BMJ. 2014;**348**:g15. DOI: 10.1136/bmj.g15

[6] Koundinya D, Anurag A. Impulse oscillometry: The state-of-art for lung function testing. Lung India. 2016;**33**:410-416. DOI: 10.4103/0970-2113.184875

[7] Jat KR, Agarwal S. Lung function tests in infants and children. Indian Journal of Pediatrics. 2023;**90**:790-797. DOI: 10.1007/s12098-023-04588-8

[8] Hoyte FCL, Gross LM, Katial RK. Exhaled nitric oxide: An update. Immunology and Allergy Clinics of North America. 2018;**38**:573-585. DOI: 10.1016/j.iac.2018.06.001

[9] Gaillard EA, Kuehni CE, Turner S, Goutaki M, Holden KA, de Jong CCM, et al. European Respiratory Society clinical practice guidelines for the diagnosis of asthma in children aged 5-16 years. The European Respiratory Journal. 2021;**58**:2004173. DOI: 10.1183/13993003.04173-2020

[10] Saglani S, Fleming L. How to manage a child with difficult asthma? Expert Review of Respiratory Medicine. 2016;**10**:873-879. DOI: 10.1080/17476348.2016.1191355

[11] Pedersen S. Preschool asthma-not so easy to diagnose. Primary Care Respiratory Journal. 2007;**16**:4-6. DOI: 10.3132/pcrj.2007.00011

[12] Sly PD, Boner AL, Bjorksten B, Bush A, Custovic A, Eigenmann PA, et al. Early identification of atopy in the prediction of persistent asthma in children. Lancet. 2008;**372**:1100-1106. DOI: 10.1016/S0140-6736(08)61451-8

[13] Jartti T, Jartti L, Ruuskanen O, Söderlund-Venermo M. New respiratory viral infections. Current Opinion in Pulmonary Medicine. 2012;**18**:271-278. DOI: 10.1097/MCP.0b013e328351f8d4

[14] Martinez FD, Wright AL, Taussing LM, Holberg CJ, Halonen M, Morgan WJ, et al. Asthma and wheezing in the first six years of life. The New England Journal of Medicine. 1995;**332**:133-138. DOI: 10.1056/NEJM199501193320301

[15] Caudri D, Wijga A, Schipper CMA, Hoekstra M, Postma DS, Koppelman GH, et al. Predicting the long-term prognosis of children with symptoms suggestive of asthma at preschool age. The Journal of Allergy and Clinical Immunology. 2009;**24**:903-910. DOI: 10.1016/j.jaci.2009.06.045

[16] Tenero L, Piazza M, Piacentini G. Recurrent wheezing in children. Transl

Pediatr. 2016;**5**:31-36. DOI: 10.3978/j.issn.2224-4336.2015.12.01

[17] Skoulakis CE, Doxas PG, Papadakis CE, Proimos E, Christodoulou P, Bizakis JG, et al. Bronchoscopy for foreign body removal in children. A review and analysis of 210 cases. International Journal of Pediatric Otorhinolaryngology. 2000;**53**:143-148. DOI: 10.1016/s0165-5876(00)00324-4

[18] Kantar A, Chang AB, Shields MD, Marchant JM, Grimwood K, Grigg J, et al. ERS statement on protracted bacterial bronchitis in children. The European Respiratory Journal. 2017;**50**:1602139. DOI: 10.1183/13993003.02139-2016

[19] Di Filippo P, Scaparrotta A, Petrosino MI, Attanasi M, Di Pillo S, Chiarelli F, et al. An underestimated cause of chronic cough: The protracted bacterial bronchitis. Annals of Thoracic Medicine. 2018;**13**:7-13. DOI: 10.4103/atm.ATM_12_17

[20] Chang AB, Upham JW, Masters IB, Redding GR, Gibson PG, Marchant JM, et al. Protracted bacterial bronchitis: The last decade and the road ahead. Pediatric Pulmonology. 2016;**51**:225-242. DOI: 10.1002/ppul.23351

[21] Villanueva G, Marceniuk G, Murphy MS, Walshaw M, Cosulich R. Guideline committee. Diagnosis and management of cystic fibrosis: Summary of NICE guidance. BMJ. 2017;**359**:j4574. DOI: 10.1136/bmj.j4574

[22] Kartal Öztürk G, Eşki A, Demir E, Gülen F. Asthma-like symptom or "cystic fibrosis asthma"? Tüberküloz ve Toraks. 2021;**69**:167-176. DOI: 10.5578/tt.20219806

[23] Satırer O, Mete Yesil A, Emiralioglu N, Tugcu GD, Yalcın E, Dogru D, et al. Are view of the etiology and clinical presentation of non- cystic fibrosis bronchiectasis: A tertiary care experienceis. Respiratory Medicine. 2018;**137**:35-39. DOI: 10.1016/j.rmed.2018.02.013

[24] Gallucci M, Di Palmo E, Bertelli L, Camela F, Ricci G, Pession A. A pediatric disease to keep in mind: Diagnostic tools and management of bronchiectasis in pediatric age. Italian Journal of Pediatrics. 2017;**43**:117. DOI: 10.1186/s13052-017-0434-0

[25] Lobo J, Zariwala MA, Noone PG. Primary ciliary dyskinesia. Seminars in Respiratory and Critical Care Medicine. 2015;**36**:169-179. DOI: 10.1055/s-0035-1546748

[26] Hazari YM, Bashir A, Habib M, Bashir S, Habib H, Qasim MA, et al. Alpha-1-antitrypsin deficiency: Genetic variations, clinical manifestations and therapeutic interventions. Mutation Research. 2017;**773**:14-25. DOI: 10.1016/j.mrrev.2017.03.001

[27] Fischer GB, Sarria EE, Mattiello R, Mocelin HT, Castro-Rodriguez JA. Post infectious bronchiolitis obliterans in children. Paediatric Respiratory Reviews. 2010;**11**:233-239. DOI: 10.1016/j.prrv.2010.07.005

[28] Enzer KG, Baker CD, Wisniewski BL. Bronchopulmonary dysplasia. Clinics in Chest Medicine. 2024;**45**:639-650. DOI: 10.1016/j.ccm.2024.03.007

[29] Hysinger EB. Laryngomalacia, tracheomalacia and bronchomalacia. Current Problems in Pediatric and Adolescent Health Care. 2018;**48**:113-118. DOI: 10.1016/j.cppeds.2018.03.002

[30] Fraga JC, Jennings RW, Kim PC. Pediatric tracheomalacia. Seminars in Pediatric Surgery. 2016;**25**:156-164. DOI: 10.1053/j.sempedsurg.2016.02.008

[31] Gormley PK, Colreavy MP, Patil N, Woods AE. Congenital vascular anomalies and persistent respiratory symptoms in children. International Journal of Pediatric Otorhinolaryngology. 1999;**51**:23-31. DOI: 10.1016/s0165-5876(99)00252-9

[32] Holbrook JT, Wise RA, Gold BD, Blake K, Brown ED, Castro M, et al. Lansoprazole for children with poorly controlled asthma: A randomized controlled trial. Journal of the American Medical Association. 2012;**307**:373-381. DOI: 10.1001/jama.2011.2035

[33] Boulet LP. Influence of comorbid conditions on asthma. The European Respiratory Journal. 2009;**33**:897-906. DOI: 10.1183/09031936.00121308

[34] Brown RW, Hanrahan JP, Castile RG, Tager IB. Effect of maternal smoking during pregnancy on passive respiratory mechanics in early in fancy. Pediatric Pulmonology. 1995;**19**:23-28. DOI: 10.1002/ppul.1950190105

[35] Marais BJ. Tuberculosis in children. Journal of Paediatrics and Child Health. 2014;**50**:759-767. DOI: 10.1111/jpc.12503

[36] Mao W, Gao Y, Sun W, Li J, Wang J, Wang Z, et al. Clinical characteristics of 31 patients with chest pain variant asthma. Journal of Asthma and Allergy. 2025;**18**:173-182. DOI: 10.2147/JAA.S494385

[37] Low K, Ruane L, Uddin N, Finlay P, Lau KK, Hamza K, et al. Abnormal vocal cord movement in patients with and without airway obstruction and asthma symptoms. Clinical and Experimental Allergy. 2017;**47**:200-207. DOI: 10.1111/cea.12828

[38] Dunn NM, Katial RK, Hoyte FCL. Vocal cord dysfunction: A review. Asthma Research and Practice. 2015;**1**:9. DOI: 10.1186/s40733-015-0009-z

[39] Yazdani R, Abolhassani H, Asgardoon M, Shaghaghi M, Modaresi M, Azizi G, et al. Infectious and noninfectious pulmonary complications in patients with primary immunodeficiency disorders. Journal of Investigational Allergology & Clinical Immunology. 2017;**27**:231-224. DOI: 10.18176/jiaci.0166

Chapter 9

Differential Diagnosis of Adult Asthma

Guzin Ozden and Leyla Cevirme

Abstract

In asthma, careful history, physical examination, and detection of variable airway obstruction in respiratory function tests provide the diagnosis. Differential diagnosis may change in childhood and adulthood. Therefore, history and examination are necessary according to age groups. It should not be forgotten that asthma can interact with many diseases, in which case diagnosis becomes difficult, and determination of asthma severity and control may be difficult. However, many diseases included in the differential diagnosis can be distinguished by radiological, histopathological, and clinical history. There are some conditions (such as allergic bronchopulmonary aspergillosis (ABPA) and eosinophilic granulomatosis with polyangiitis (EGPA)) where asthma is a component of these diseases, and instead of differentiating, it is necessary to define other accompanying system findings. Taking a careful history can help distinguish some diseases, such as drug-related cough and gastroesophageal reflux, from asthma without the need for diagnostic tests. Again, some diseases begin in childhood and are based on genetics. It may be relatively easy to distinguish these diseases from asthma.

Keywords: asthma, differential diagnosis, EGPA, ABPA, COPD, CF, chronic cough

1. Introduction

1.1. The diseases included in the differential diagnosis and their characteristics

Asthma is an airway disease characterized by chronic airway inflammation and remodeling. It is a disease in which eosinophils and mast cells play an important role, but many cells and mediators are also involved. Symptoms include shortness of breath, wheezing, cough, and chest discomfort, usually with morning attacks. Asthma can be diagnosed by spirometry, and reversible airway obstruction supports the diagnosis. Chronic cough, a common symptom, is particularly important in the differential diagnosis of asthma. With all these clinical and symptomatic features, asthma can be confused with many lung diseases.

2. Chronic upper airway cough syndrome

Upper airway cough syndrome (UACS) is caused by the depletion of nasal secretions flowing into the nasopharynx; therefore, one of the most common causes of chronic cough was formerly known as "postnasal drip syndrome." Other common causes of chronic cough are asthma and gastroesophageal reflux disease. The primary etiologies of Upper Airway Cough Syndrome (UACS) are categorised as allergic, perennial, non-allergic, and vasomotor rhinitis, in addition to rhinosinusitis. Diagnosis of UACS is based on clinical exclusion, as there is no diagnostic test or objective finding. Diagnosis is confirmed by resolution of symptoms following therapeutic intervention [1, 2].

The pathogenesis of cough in UACS may be multifactorial. Triggers such as mechanical or chemical stimuli in the peripheral sensory terminals of the trigeminal nerve and upper branches of the vagus nerve may cause coughing. According to the airway hypothesis, inflammatory mediators spread hematogenously and neurally between the upper and lower airways. When secretions are present in the upper respiratory tract, a cough is likely triggered by stimulation of cough receptors in the laryngeal mucosa [3].

Common symptoms include sneezing, nasal itching, congestion, rhinorrhea, postnasal drip, and persistent throat clearing [4]. However, symptomatic absence does not definitively exclude the diagnosis. Nasopharyngeal examination may reveal a cobblestone appearance of the pharyngeal mucosa or pharyngeal secretions. Given the nonspecific nature of sinus mucosal thickening on imaging, radiographic evaluation is typically reserved for cases refractory to empiric chronic rhinitis therapy [2].

UACS, which is in the differential diagnosis of chronic cough and asthma, should be investigated. Although the diagnostic criteria are not clear, the patient can be excluded by evaluating the results of clinical examination and tests.

3. Airway foreign bodies in adults

Foreign body aspiration (FBA) is a more prevalent condition in children than in adults. In adults, the condition is characterized by an insidious onset of a persistent cough, often overlooked due to the absence of discernible imaging findings. The diagnosis of this condition is often delayed, as it necessitates a high index of clinical suspicion on the part of the treating physician. Definitive diagnosis usually requires direct visualization of the foreign body during bronchoscopy. In adults, key risk factors encompass trauma, drug or alcohol intoxication, and anesthesia-induced loss of consciousness. Conversely, elderly populations face additional risks, including age-related swallowing dysfunction, polypharmacy, poststroke dysphagia, and neurodegenerative disorders such as Alzheimer's and Parkinson's diseases [5].

Symptom presentation varies according to the site of obstruction. Chronic cough due to distal lower airway obstruction is often followed by symptoms that mimic pneumonia, such as fever, chest pain, and hemoptysis. Rarely, acute asphyxia occurs with acute symptoms of upper airway obstruction (stridor or choking) in adults due to large obstructive upper respiratory tract foreign bodies. Fever, hemoptysis, foul-smelling sputum, chest pain, or wheezing are detectable symptoms [6]. Generally, foreign bodies are aspirated into the lower lobes and cause distal bronchial obstruction. The right bronchus is the most common site of aspiration because the right main bronchus has a more vertical angle and sometimes a slightly larger diameter than the left.

It is important to note that long-standing foreign bodies have been known to mimic both benign and malignant diseases. For example, unexplained dyspnea or unilateral wheezing may occur, mimicking the symptoms of atypical asthma. Furthermore, a foreign body may be incidentally detected during flexible bronchoscopy performed for diseases and symptoms such as chronic cough, hemoptysis, and asthma that do not respond to treatment, or recurrent/unresolved pneumonia. Therefore, although this condition is comparatively rare in adults, it should be considered in cases where children are affected.

4. Heart failure

Heart failure (HF) has been identified as the foremost global cause of death, morbidity, and poor quality of life. The clinical syndrome is characterized by symptoms and/or signs resulting from structural and/or functional cardiac abnormalities. These abnormalities are confirmed by elevated levels of natriuretic peptides and/or objective evidence of pulmonary or systemic congestion [7].

In pulmonary edema, a nonproductive cough results from airway edema and mucosal irritation, whereas a productive cough with frothy sputum reflects alveolar fluid accumulation. Characteristic signs of heart failure—including peripheral edema, auscultatory abnormalities, elevated jugular venous pressure, ascites, pleural effusion, and pulmonary vascular redistribution—are typically present and serve to distinguish this condition from asthma.

Asthma is a prevalent etiology of chronic cough in adults, characterized by episodic wheezing and dyspnea. Conversely, the presence of symptoms such as orthopnea, paroxysmal nocturnal dyspnea, cardiac arrhythmias, peripheral edema, a prior cardiac history, auscultatory crackles, and elevated jugular venous pressure is associated with heart failure. The diagnostic workup should include electrocardiography, BNP measurement, cardiac biomarkers, chest radiography, and echocardiography when indicated.

5. Inducible laryngeal obstruction

Inducible laryngeal obstruction (ILO) is characterized by transient, reversible laryngeal narrowing in response to triggering stimuli. Under normal physiological conditions, the vocal folds abduct during inspiration and exhibit slight adduction during expiration, coughing, and phonation. During ILO episodes, paradoxical vocal fold adduction may occur during either inspiration, expiration, or both phases of respiration. The term ILO is clinically preferred to "paradoxical vocal fold movement" as it encompasses the dynamic airway narrowing that may involve both the false vocal folds and supraglottic structures. While frequently misdiagnosed as asthma, ILO may coexist with asthma. The presence of diagnostic confusion is attributable to the manifestation of shared features, which include the occurrence of episodic symptoms, the presentation of symptoms induced by exercise, and acoustic characteristics that are analogous (e.g., stridor in ILO versus expiratory wheezing in asthma). Bronchoconstriction (e.g., during histamine-induced breathing difficulty) may sometimes trigger or coexist with laryngeal obstruction in patients [8]. Although laryngoscopy is usually normal between attacks, laryngoscopy performed during symptomatic attacks is the gold standard for diagnosis [9].

Diagnostic features supporting asthma (with or without concomitant ILO) include demonstration of reversible airflow obstruction on spirometry and clinical improvement with appropriate asthma therapy. Laryngoscopic findings may reveal expiratory vocal cord adduction, which in some asthma patients represents a form of intrinsic positive end-expiratory pressure. This phenomenon typically resolves with adequate asthma control [10, 11].

6. Hyperventilation syndrome in adults

Hyperventilation syndrome is characterized by diverse symptomatology without identifiable organic pathology, leading to respiratory alkalosis through excessive minute ventilation disproportionate to metabolic demand. Considerable debate persists regarding its etiology, diagnostic criteria, and therapeutic management. Although extant research has established a frequent association between hyperventilation episodes and panic disorder, it is important to note that other precipitating factors may also contribute significantly to the etiology of the condition. Dysfunctional breathing is another term used for a condition like hyperventilation syndrome. For transient increase in minute ventilation, lasting from a few minutes to an hour and resolving spontaneously, hyperventilation episodes usually resolve without complications. Symptoms are dyspnea, dizziness, chest pain or tightness, paresthesia, and palpitations [12]. In patients with hyperventilation syndrome, symptoms often occur with unpredictable frequency and intermittency.

Hyperventilation syndrome is characterized by diverse symptomatology without identifiable organic pathology, leading to respiratory alkalosis through excessive minute ventilation disproportionate to metabolic demand. Considerable debate persists regarding its etiology, diagnostic criteria, and therapeutic management. While evidence establishes a frequent association between hyperventilation episodes and panic disorder, other precipitating factors may contribute significantly.

However, for patients presenting with acute hyperventilation, the differential diagnosis of not only asthma but also a range of respiratory, cardiac, metabolic, and infectious diseases becomes challenging.

7. Gastroesophageal reflux disease (GERD)

Gastroesophageal reflux is a condition that can be seen in healthy people, but to be called a disease, stomach acid, and/or bile-containing stomach content must leak back into the esophagus, and the esophagus must not be able to protect itself from the acid and/or bile-containing stomach content after this contact, and complaints must occur accordingly. The pathophysiology of GERD and asthma can be explained by the physiological mechanisms that mediate the causal relationship between the two diseases, the "reflux" and "reflex" theories. In the reflux theory, passage of gastric contents into the lower respiratory tract directly damages the epithelium, causing inflammation through cytokine release. Acidification of the airway epithelium can induce nitric oxide synthesis, eosinophil necrosis, decreased ciliary movement, and increased airway mucosal viscosity. Studies have also shown that gastric acid leakage into the airways increases bronchial hyperresponsiveness and reduces peak expiratory flow [13].

Chronic cough, recurrent bronchitis, pneumonia, and asthma attacks are associated with reflux disease. If there is no improvement in asthma-related complaints despite effective asthma treatment, if the patient's cough continues, and if the patient's complaints of shortness of breath at night continue, it should be considered that there may be an underlying reflux problem. In asthma patients, stomach acid due to reflux can increase asthma attacks by stimulating the bronchi. It is imperative to consider this as both a differential diagnosis for asthma and a triggering factor in refractory asthma cases, despite the presence of adequate treatment [14].

8. Eosinophilic granulomatosis with polyangiitis (EGPA)

Eosinophilic granulomatosis with polyangiitis (EGPA) is characterized by granulomatous and eosinophil-rich inflammation and systemic necrotizing vasculitis affecting small- to medium-sized vessels, evolving in three sequential phases: allergic, eosinophilic, and vasculitic phases [15].

The diagnostic criteria for eosinophilic granulomatosis with polyangiitis (EGPA), as defined by the American College of Rheumatology (ACR), include a peripheral blood eosinophil count exceeding 10% or an absolute eosinophil count greater than 1000 cells/mm^3, in conjunction with asthma, and the presence of at least two of the following features: histopathological evidence of eosinophilic vasculitis, perivascular eosinophilic infiltration, or granulomatous inflammation with marked eosinophilic involvement; non-fixed pulmonary infiltrates identified *via* imaging; chronic sinonasal disease, particularly chronic rhinosinusitis with nasal polyposis (CRSwNP); and peripheral neuropathy, which may present as mononeuropathy or polyneuropathy with motor deficits, or be confirmed by abnormal nerve conduction studies [16].

The exact pathogenesis of EGPA is unknown. Although eosinophilic granulomatosis with polyangiitis (EGPA) is classified as an ANCA-associated vasculitis, only 30–40% of patients test positive for antineutrophil cytoplasmic antibodies (ANCA) [17].

Eosinophils, increased in EGPA, initiate the production of cytokines and are considered important in producing tissue fibrosis, as shown in endomyocardial fibrosis and airway remodeling in EGPA patients. Differences in EGPA phenotypes may be observed according to ANCA positivity. While positive patients exhibit vasculitis with peripheral neuropathy, progressive glomerulonephritis, gastrointestinal findings, and multiorgan involvement, cardiomyopathy, which is one of the major eosinophil-induced complications, is observed in ANCA-negative patients [18]. Detection of other findings accompanying respiratory complaints leads to the diagnosis of EGPA rather than asthma.

9. Alpha-1 antitrypsin deficiency

Alpha-1 antitrypsin deficiency (AATD) is an inherited, autosomal dominant disease affecting the lungs, liver, and occasionally the skin. Deficiency of AAT in the lungs causes chronic obstructive pulmonary disease (emphysema and bronchiectasis). Dyspnea is the most common symptom, and many patients report chronic sputum production and wheezing. Bronchodilator sensitivity has been defined by older criteria as a 200 mL or 12% increase in postbronchodilator forced expiratory volume in 1 second (FEV 1) or, more recently, a change of >10% from predicted FEV 1 or forced vital capacity (FVC) [19].

Features that specifically warrant testing for AATD include age < 45 years, emphysema in a nonsmoker or light smoker, emphysema characterized by predominant basilar changes on chest radiograph, liver disease, family history, panniculitis, and persistent airflow obstruction on postbronchodilator spirometry.

10. *Bordetella pertussis*

Pertussis (also known as whooping cough) is a highly infectious disease caused by the bacterium *Bordetella pertussis* and characterized by an acute respiratory infection. There are three clinical phases of whooping cough disease, respectively: the catarrhal phase, the paroxysmal phase, and the recovery phase.

The catarrhal phase manifests with nonspecific systemic symptoms, including malaise, rhinorrhea, mild cough, and low-grade fever, which typically persist for 1–2 weeks. This phase is followed by the paroxysmal stage. The hallmark symptom, paroxysmal cough, is a severe, consecutive cough that occurs during a single exhalation. After a prolonged cough, a violent inhalation causes a "whooping" sound due to the small caliber of the trachea. Cough can occur regardless of day or night. Although they feel comfortable between coughing attacks, they can be triggered by laughing, yawning, shouting, and exercise. Sometimes syncope or vomiting may also occur after coughing. This period may last 1–2 months before recovery. The recovery phase usually lasts 1 to 2 weeks, although it can be prolonged. The frequency and severity of the cough gradually decrease.

Pertussis represents a prevalent yet frequently underdiagnosed etiology of chronic cough in adolescent and adult populations. Clinical studies demonstrate significantly prolonged diagnostic delays in adult cases compared to pediatric patients [20]. Clinical manifestations of pertussis in adolescents and adults are less severe than in children, and sometimes a prolonged cough may be the only symptom [21]. According to the United States Centers for Disease Control and Prevention and the World Health Organization, it is defined as a cough lasting at least 2 weeks without any obvious cause, accompanied by at least one of the following features: cough attacks, inspiratory cough, or post-cough vomiting [22].

11. Bronchiectasis

Radiologically, bronchiectasis is defined as persistent dilatation of the bronchi, while clinically it is defined as coughing, producing sputum, and experiencing recurrent lung infections [23, 24]. In 2013, the prevalence of bronchiectasis was reported to have increased by 40% since 2003, reaching 566 per 100,000 people [25]. The pathophysiology of bronchiectasis is explained by the "vicious cycle" model. Impaired mucociliary clearance in dilated bronchi leads to the buildup of secretions, which makes the airway susceptible to chronic bacterial infection. This, in turn, triggers an inflammatory response, causing abnormal airway remodeling and structural damage [26]. Interrupting the cycle by intervening with one of the components—abnormal mucus, chronic infection, or inflammation—may lead to a positive clinical outcome. Bronchiectasis is known to be a complication of asthma and has been reported in up to 50% of patients with severe asthma on high-resolution computed tomography (HRCT) scans [27, 28].

However, bronchiectasis is also considered a separate disease with a different definition and diagnostic criteria [23].

The diagnostic complexity of asthma and bronchiectasis is that patients with bronchiectasis as the primary diagnosis have chronic airway inflammation and asthma-like respiratory symptoms and may present with airflow obstruction [29]. Bronchiectasis has generally been considered a neutrophilic disorder, whereas asthma has been associated with predominantly eosinophilic inflammation. The recognition of neutrophilic subtypes of asthma and eosinophilic subtypes of bronchiectasis further complicates the distinction between these conditions [30, 31].

Patients with bronchiectasis without a diagnosis of asthma often have sensitization to environmental allergens and elevated T helper 2 (TH2) inflammatory markers, which have been associated with an increased risk of asthma exacerbations [30, 32].

Bronchiectasis is a clinical condition that causes airway obstruction, anatomical defects in the airway, disorders in host defense, some rheumatological diseases, ciliary dyskinesias, and frequent pulmonary infections. It is also a component of the disease in allergic bronchopulmonary aspergillosis (ABPA), asthma, Young syndrome (bronchiectasis, sinusitis, and obstructive azoospermia), and cystic fibrosis (CF). As a result of spirometry, obstructive pathology is seen in bronchiectasis, but a decrease in FVC and an increase in residual volume (RV) may be observed [33].

Since respiratory symptoms seen in both asthma and bronchiectasis are common, clinical findings alone are not sufficient for differentiation. However, since bronchiectasis usually occurs after another pulmonary infection or together with some diseases (ABPA, Young Syndrome, etc.), it can be differentiated from asthma with clinical history. Radiological findings seen in bronchiectasis (dilated bronchi, signet ring appearance, train track appearance, saccular bronchus appearance, etc.) are often not observed in asthma. Asthma is diagnosed with spirometry, which shows deterioration in respiratory function. Almost always, the ratio of FEV1 to FVC is low, the FEV1 ratio is low, and the FVC is normal. In addition, an airway reversibility that responds to beta 2 agonists is detected. However, none of these may be present in bronchiectasis, and FEV1, FVC, and/or RV may be increased. Airway reversibility may be absent.

12. Chronic obstructive pulmonary disease

Chronic obstructive pulmonary disease (COPD) is a heterogeneous inflammatory lung disorder characterized by chronic respiratory symptoms (dyspnea, cough, sputum production, and/or exacerbations) due to abnormalities in the airways and/or alveoli. This condition causes persistent, usually progressive airflow limitation [34].

The primary exposures that cause COPD are tobacco smoking and inhalation of toxic particles and gases from indoor and/or outdoor air pollution. Other environmental and host factors (including abnormal lung development and accelerated lung aging) may also contribute [35–37]. The diagnosis of COPD is confirmed by spirometric demonstration of fully reversible airflow limitation, defined as a post-bronchodilator FEV1/FVC ratio < 0.7. However, certain individuals exhibit structural lung abnormalities and/or physiological impairments despite maintaining a post-bronchodilator FEV1/FVC ratio ≥ 0.7. This clinical phenotype may be classified as "Pre-COPD."

COPD typically manifests with dyspnea, wheezing, chest tightness, fatigue, activity limitation, and/or chronic cough. A hallmark of the disease is acute exacerbations, defined by worsening respiratory symptoms that may include increased sputum production. These exacerbations significantly impact both health status and long-term prognosis. Importantly, COPD patients frequently exhibit comorbid conditions that influence disease progression and clinical outcomes, necessitating targeted management. Such comorbidities may clinically mimic or potentiate acute exacerbations [38].

Asthma and chronic obstructive pulmonary disease (COPD) represent two prevalent chronic respiratory disorders characterized by persistent airflow limitation and consequent dyspnea, both involving chronic inflammatory processes of the respiratory mucosa. Despite these similarities, they are fundamentally distinct entities with divergent risk factors, clinical trajectories, pathophysiological mechanisms, therapeutic responses, and associated comorbidities.

Asthma, frequently associated with atopy, typically manifests in childhood (though onset may occur at any age). It is characterized by variable airflow obstruction, airway hyperresponsiveness, and type 2 predominant inflammation, featuring eosinophilic infiltration and mast cell activation within the airway mucosa. In contrast, COPD demonstrates adult-onset, progressive airflow limitation; predominant association with chronic exposure to noxious particles (particularly cigarette smoke); neutrophil-mediated inflammation, primarily affecting small airways and lung parenchyma. Notably, some patients exhibit overlapping features of both conditions. Additionally, each syndrome encompasses multiple distinct endotypes and phenotypes that warrant clinical recognition [39].

Patients with features of asthma and COPD may be referred to as the "asthma-COPD overlap syndrome"; however, recognizing that this overlap condition has heterogeneous aspects, these patients have recently been labeled asthma-COPD overlap (ACO) [40].

Episodic symptoms are seen in asthma, while symptoms are progressive in COPD. In addition, there is reversible airway limitation with asthmatic bronchial hyperresponsiveness. In COPD, this reversible airway limitation may not always be detected. Once more, while eosinophils and mast cells are present in cases of asthma due to inflammation, neutrophilic infiltration and less eosinophilic inflammation are detected in cases of COPD. Therefore, the response to corticosteroids is better in asthma. Although eosinophils are the predominant cell in asthma, an increase in neutrophil count is detected in the sputum of a group of patients. It has been demonstrated that these patients are typically smokers, and their response to corticosteroids is reduced. The resultant effect of this is that more severe asthma and lower lung function are observed [41].

Elevated blood eosinophil counts (≥300 cells/μL) are a biomarker that is usually linked to asthma. This is seen in a group of COPD patients. This eosinophilic phenotype demonstrates distinct clinical characteristics, including increased exacerbation frequency, greater bronchodilator responsiveness, and accelerated lung function decline [42].

Eosinophilic COPD may represent a different endotype of COPD or may represent concurrent asthma in a COPD patient, making it difficult to distinguish between the two diseases. Triple inhalers containing two long-acting bronchodilators and a corticosteroid have seen a marked increase in utilization in recent years. These triple inhalers treat both diseases and have been found to be useful [40].

However, corticosteroids are the basis of treatment in asthma. In COPD, corticosteroids are considered only in patients with a high number of exacerbations, high dyspnea scores, and low exercise capacity. Therefore, the distinction between the two diseases should be made from the very beginning of the disease. Moreover, early-onset asthma—often associated with atopic diseases (e.g., allergic rhinitis, nasal polyps, or atopic dermatitis), eosinophilia, and a positive family history—may help differentiate between these two conditions. It may not always be possible to distinguish based on spirometry and radiology results. However, radiological differentiation may be useful in COPD patients with emphysema.

13. Pulmonary embolism

Pulmonary embolism (PE) occurs due to blockage of a pulmonary artery or one or more of its branches by material (e.g., thrombus, tumor, air, or fat) formed elsewhere in the body. PE is an acute/subacute disease with nonspecific symptoms and findings, frequently diagnosed in emergency departments. The estimated annual incidence is 39–115 per 100,000 people. Classic risk factors for the development of this disease include major trauma, lower extremity surgery, previous venous thromboembolism, recent hospitalization, use of oral contraception, postpartum period, malignancy, and thrombophilia. The disease can be fatal. Recent studies have found that mortality associated with PE is 1–3%. Symptoms of PE may include chest pain, dyspnea, cough, syncope, or hemoptysis. These symptoms are nonspecific, and, as a result, a suspected diagnosis of PE typically requires a clinical assessment of probability and potentially D-dimer testing and/or imaging [43].

Pulmonary angiographic CT is the preferred imaging method for diagnosis in high-risk patients or in patients with clinical suspicion of PE and elevated D-dimer levels; the examinations are highly sensitive and specific for diagnosis [44].

Ventilation-perfusion scintigraphy may be helpful for diagnosis, especially in the presence of thrombus affecting subsegmental pulmonary artery branches, in subacute or chronic conditions. Treatment is planned according to the clinical classification made together with risk and diagnostic methods (echocardiography, CTPA, D-dimer, etc.). Thrombolytic agents, oral/subcutaneous/intravenous anticoagulants, and supportive treatment may be given in the treatment. Patients are treated with or without hospitalization according to the clinical classification. Clinical findings in PE are mostly acute in onset, and a predisposing risk factor is needed for its development. Asthma encompasses a patient population that, while not in acute status, may remain entirely asymptomatic between episodic exacerbations. While it is possible to distinguish acute and subacute PE from asthma with clinical findings, it may be difficult to distinguish chronic thromboembolic disease. In this case, ventilation perfusion scintigraphy and echocardiography (ECHO) are diagnostic tests in favor of PE. Obstruction and/or reversible airway stenosis with beta2 agonist on spirometry may diagnose asthma.

14. Diffuse parenchymal lung diseases

Interstitial lung disease (diffuse parenchymal diseases) is a heterogeneous group of diseases characterized by fibrosis (scarring) of the lungs. They are classified according to histopathological, radiological, and clinical parameters [45].

Diffuse parenchymal lung diseases (DPLD) are classified into two distinct categories: those with identifiable etiologies and idiopathic forms. Both therapeutic approaches and clinical outcomes vary significantly across the spectrum of interstitial lung diseases (ILD), depending on their underlying pathogenesis and disease subtype.

Diffuse parenchymal lung diseases manifest radiologically as interstitial opacities with diverse etiologies, broadly categorized into infectious and noninfectious causes. It is widely acknowledged that the most significant identifiable causes of ILD include occupational and environmental exposures (inorganic/organic particulates), drug-induced pulmonary toxicity, and radiation pneumonitis. A significant subset of ILD cases develops as pulmonary complications of connective tissue diseases, including rheumatoid arthritis, systemic sclerosis, inflammatory myopathies, and mixed connective tissue disease, where its presence adversely impacts disease prognosis. The idiopathic interstitial pneumonias (encompassing idiopathic pulmonary fibrosis and nonspecific interstitial pneumonia), cryptogenic organizing pneumonia, and sarcoidosis constitute important diagnostic entities when no underlying etiology is identified. Progressive dyspnea and persistent cough may be observed in patients with ILD. The potential causes of non-idiopathic ILD, such as medication use, connective tissue disease, and occupational exposure, should be thoroughly investigated. Radiological changes are almost always detected in ILD. Spirometry and carbon monoxide diffusion tests (DLCO) are used in diagnosis [46]. .Lung function assessment has a crucial role in the diagnosis, prognosis, and treatment of ILD. Not only in initial diagnosis but also in follow-up and prognosis [47] patients suffering from ILD who present with low FVC and DLCO at the baseline face an elevated risk of mortality [48]. With all these features, it is not very difficult to distinguish ILD from asthma. In asthma, if it is not complicated by infection or pneumothorax, there is often no radiographic finding. In spirometry, there is almost always a reversible decrease in FEV1 and a normal FVC. A decrease in DLCO is not expected. In asthma, shortness of breath is not chronically progressive; it occurs in attacks, usually at night toward morning, and the patient can be completely normal between attacks. Other system findings accompanying asthma, other than comorbidities, are not expected. However, organ-specific symptoms can be seen in the presence of rhinitis, nasal polyps, or EGPA. On physical examination, hearing rales is not typical for asthma and suggests another accompanying pathology, such as heart failure. Bronchial rhonchi can be heard during attacks or when the patient is symptomatic. While treatment for ILD is based on the etiology, corticosteroids or immunosuppressive agents are used; asthma is treated with inhaled corticosteroids and symptom-relieving agents (such as beta-2 agonists).

15. Allergic bronchopulmonary aspergillosis (ABPA)

Allergic bronchopulmonary aspergillosis (ABPA) is a chronic lung disease involving hypersensitivity to *Aspergillus fumigatus*. The condition is often linked to high levels of total IgE in the blood and positive *A. fumigatus*-specific IgE/IgG antibodies. ABPA primarily affects individuals with asthma or cystic fibrosis [49]. Patients with ABPA typically present with respiratory symptoms such as wheezing, mucus plugging, pulmonary infiltrates, and occasionally systemic symptoms. ABPA may complicate asthma (2.5% prevalence) and cystic fibrosis (7.8% prevalence) [50].

Histological features of ABPA are consistent with asthma, including mucoid impaction of the bronchi, eosinophilic pneumonia, and bronchocentric granulomatosis. While focal areas of eosinophilic pneumonia may be observed, these do not represent a dominant pathological feature. The precise pathogenesis of ABPA remains incompletely elucidated, though T lymphocytes, particularly *Aspergillus* antigen-specific Th2 CD4+ cells, play a pivotal role in both bronchial-associated lymphoid tissue and systemic circulation. These antigen-responsive T cells activate eosinophils in peripheral blood and airways while promoting the secretion of Th2 cytokines (IL-4, IL-5, IL-13), thereby driving immunoglobulin E (IgE) overproduction. Aspergillus colonization of the asthmatic airways elicits a strong IgE- and IgG-mediated immune response. Despite robust immune responses in ABPA, *Aspergillus* species persist in airway colonization, precipitating recurrent symptomatology. Fungal-derived proteolytic enzymes and mycotoxins—acting in concert with Th2-driven eosinophilic inflammation and IL-8-mediated neutrophilic recruitment—collectively contribute to airway epithelial injury and the development of central bronchiectasis [51]. The clinical picture of ABPA is asthmatic and recurrent exacerbations. In severe cases, there may be bronchial obstruction, fever, malaise, expectoration of brown mucus plugs, and occasionally hemoptysis. Exacerbations (usually symptomatic exacerbations characterized by shortness of breath, wheezing, and increased sputum production) cause a decline in lung function [52]. Some patients with ABPA develop allergic *Aspergillus rhinosinusitis* with pulmonary manifestations. This condition manifests clinically as nasal congestion, sinus pressure, and viscous rhinorrhea [53].

The diagnosis is based on a set of criteria updated by the International Society of Human and Animal Mycology (ISHAM) in 2024. They established a diagnostic criterion based on the presence of two mandatory criteria (high *Aspergillus*-specific; IgE ≥ 0.35 kUA L^{-1} and high total IgE levels; ≥500 IU mL^{-1}) and the presence of two of three secondary criteria (high *Aspergillus*-specific IgG levels, presence of eosinophilia in the blood: ≥500 cells μL^{-1}, and compatible radiological findings bronchiectasis, mucus plugging, and high-attenuation mucus) [54]. If left untreated, ABPA can lead to recurrent exacerbations, development of central bronchiectasis, fibro-cavitary lung disease, poor quality of life, and eventually death. Twenty-five to 50% of patients experience an exacerbation after discontinuation of initial therapy. Additionally, 20–45% of patients become glucocorticoid dependent for long-term management of their ABPA [55].

HRCT is the gold standard for the diagnosis of bronchiectasis. Bronchiectasis in ABPA can affect any region of the lung but most commonly affects the upper and middle lobes and the central bronchi. Bronchiectasis presents as ring shadows or parallel linear opacities (trolley line sign). Mucoid impaction results in tubular or branching opacities (gloved finger sign). Bronchial obstruction may result in atelectasis or obstructive pneumonitis and may present radiographically. Transient opacities, bronchiectasis, and mucoid impaction and findings associated with bronchial obstruction may also be seen on imaging [56].

Many patients exhibit characteristic pulmonary function abnormalities, including airflow obstruction, air trapping, reduced FEV1, and elevated residual volume. A study of patient outcomes reveals that fewer than half of patients exhibit a positive bronchodilator response. A mixed obstructive and restrictive pattern may be observed in individuals diagnosed with bronchiectasis or fibrosis. A small number of patients have decreased diffusing capacity, an abnormality that may be more common in the presence of bronchiectasis [51].

The prevailing evidence for the treatment and management of ABPA is primarily based on oral corticosteroids (OCS) or azole antifungal therapy, which are used in the initial management of patients. Itraconazole and voriconazole are indicated as monotherapy for the treatment of acute ABPA; however, these medications are frequently utilized as adjunctive or steroid-sparing therapy in patients diagnosed with glucocorticoid-dependent ABPA. The utilization of azole has been demonstrated to effectuate a reduction in corticosteroid dosage, sputum inflammatory markers, serum IgE levels, and the frequency of exacerbations [50].

ABPA occurring in the absence of asthma or cystic fibrosis represents an uncommon clinical entity. Among a cohort of 530 ABPA patients, only 37 cases (7%) manifested without underlying asthma [57].

If an asthmatic patient has a skin test reaction, especially to *Aspergillus*, then ABPA becomes a diagnostic possibility. The reported prevalence of ABPA among asthmatic populations demonstrates considerable variability. A substantial proportion of asthma patients exhibit one or more features suggestive of ABPA yet fail to fulfill complete diagnostic criteria. Serologic testing reveals *Aspergillus*-precipitating antibodies in approximately 10% of both non-ABPA asthmatics and patients with non-asthmatic chronic lung disease. Furthermore, immediate hypersensitivity skin testing demonstrates positive reactions to *A. fumigatus* antigens in 20–30% of asthmatic individuals without ABPA. ABPA is in the same disease spectrum as asthma with fungal sensitization, making it difficult to distinguish between these conditions, especially when determining the total and specific IgE values that define the disease [51, 58].

16. Cystic fibrosis (CF)

Cystic fibrosis (CF) is an autosomal recessive disease caused by mutations in the CF transmembrane conductance regulator (CFTR) gene. It is the most common lifelong genetic disease in the Caucasian population. It affects at least 100,000 people worldwide. Typical symptoms and signs include persistent pulmonary infection, pancreatic insufficiency, and high sweat chloride levels [59].

Although most people with cystic fibrosis die at a young age, life expectancy has seen considerable improvement in recent years [60]. According to data records from the Cystic Fibrosis Foundation (CFF), the median age at which people born between 2019 and 2023 can be expected to die is 61 [61].

The CFTR gene encodes a chloride ion channel that is expressed in epithelial cells in the sweat glands, lungs, pancreas, intestines, and reproductive systems, among other places. The protein is synthesized intracellularly and transported to the plasma membrane, where it controls the secretion of ions and water. To date, more than 2000 CFTR variants have been identified, each with different effects on the protein. Of these variants, pathogenic ones are generally divided into six classes. As indicated by the literature, this includes variants that alter the production of the protein (class I) and/or processing and biochemical maturation (class II), regulation of the CFTR channel (class III), chlorine (Cl^-) conductance (class IV), reduced abundance (V), and reduced stability (VI) [62]. .Individuals who carry class IV–VI variants generally exhibit milder symptoms, while those with class I–III variants tend to manifest severe disease [63]. The most prevalent CF mutation to date is the class II variant, deletion of phenylalanine 508 (F508del), which accounts for two-thirds of cases worldwide. It is evident that all identified pathogenic variants of the CFTR protein result in diminished chloride secretion. This, in turn, precipitates elevated sodium and water uptake in the pertinent anatomical regions. Increased water uptake in the airway epithelium results in thickening of the mucus layer. Thickened mucus provides an ideal environment for bacterial infections by reducing mucociliary clearance in the lung and causing bronchial obstruction. The development of chronic inflammation within the lung has been demonstrated to result in structural damage to the airways, ultimately leading to the condition known as bronchiectasis. The vicious cycle of mucus thickening, decreased clearance, and bronchiectasis results in ventilatory failure, which is the primary cause of death from cystic fibrosis. Obstructions resulting from the high viscosity of the secretions can also affect the pancreas. The secretion of pancreatic enzymes into the intestine is impaired, and there is a possibility that the enzymes may target pancreatic tissue, leading to autodigestion. It is important to note that pancreatitis and endocrine pancreatic. Decreased pancreatic bicarbonate secretion lowers the pH, which may prevent effective neutralization or digestion of sour gastric chyme. This may cause oily stools, diarrhea, and impaired nutrient absorption. Conversely, obstructions within the biliary and hepatic systems have the potential to result in gallstone formation, cirrhosis, elevated hepatic portal vein pressure, esophageal varices, splenomegaly, and hypersplenism [64]. Patients diagnosed with CF later in childhood were more likely to present with atypical symptoms. A large retrospective cohort study of over 1000 CF patients found that 7% of patients were diagnosed at ≥18 years of age. Patients diagnosed in adulthood were more likely than children to present with gastrointestinal symptoms, diabetes mellitus, and infertility. Additionally, adults presenting with CF were more likely than children to have unusual genetic mutations, normal pancreatic function, and indeterminate sweat chloride test results [65]. The diagnosis of cystic fibrosis is based on biochemical or genetic confirmation in the presence of compatible clinical findings. In most cases, sweat chloride testing is the first and most important test. DNA testing is used for confirmation or further evaluation of patients with intermediate sweat chloride results and for prognostic and epidemiological purposes in individuals with positive sweat chloride test results. Sweat testing is performed by sweat collection and chemical determination of chloride concentration with pilocarpine iontophoresis [46]. CF treatment includes CFTR modulators and specific treatments and care specific to the organ affected. Asthma is an airway disease characterized by atopic and/or eosinophilic airway inflammation, and genetic defects such as those in CF have not yet been identified. Although both diseases appear to have similar clinical symptoms of cough and shortness of breath, they are different entities. CF is clearly distinguishable from asthma because it is a genetic disease that is usually diagnosed in the neonatal period, involves extrapulmonary pathologies, and can result in mortality.

17. Medication-related cough

Cough is a complex reflex involving coordination between various muscles and nerve pathways. Cough is a protective mechanism for the respiratory system. It helps to clear the airways of substances that can damage or interfere with normal breathing. Cough can be categorized into three distinct classifications based on the duration of symptoms: acute, subacute, and chronic cough. Chronic cough (CC) is defined as a persistent cough that persists for a duration of 8 weeks or more in adults. Subacute cough is characterized as a duration of 3 to 8 weeks, while acute cough is typically defined as a duration of less than 3 weeks. CC is a condition that has the potential to have a considerable impact on quality of life and can present a diagnostic challenge [66].

Chronic cough phenotypes include upper airway cough syndrome, rhinitis and rhinosinusitis, obstructive sleep apnea syndrome, laryngeal hypersensitivity, lower airway cough syndrome, reflux-related cough, acute eosinophilic bronchitis, chronic bronchitis, coughs due to medications, malignancies, and interstitial lung diseases. Cough represents a well-documented adverse effect of multiple pharmacologic classes, particularly angiotensin-converting enzyme (ACE) inhibitors. Drug cessation serves both diagnostic and therapeutic purposes, with symptom resolution typically occurring within several days following discontinuation of the offending agent.

A nonproductive cough represents a well-characterized adverse effect associated with ACE inhibitor therapy [2]. It is more common in women than men, and also more common in Chinese Patients [67]. ACE inhibitors are postulated to enhance cough reflex sensitivity, likely mediated through bradykinin accumulation—a substrate normally metabolized by ACE that stimulates airway C-fiber afferents. A characteristic nonproductive cough develops in 5–20% of ACE inhibitor-treated patients, typically emerging within 1–2 weeks of therapy initiation but potentially persisting for 6 months. Women are more frequently affected than men. It resolves within 1 to 4 days after stopping treatment but may take up to 4 weeks. It usually recurs when the same or a different ACE inhibitor is used again. It is not more common in asthmatic patients but may be associated with bronchospasm. It is not yet clear why cough occurs only in some patients treated with ACE inhibitors. It has been suggested that genetic factors may be important. In a genetic study of approximately 80,000 individuals treated with ACE inhibitors, discontinuation of treatment due to cough was associated with seven loci; these loci were also associated with gastroesophageal reflux disease, allergic rhinitis, and asthma [68]. Pharmacologic agents that exacerbate gastroesophageal reflux—including calcium channel blockers and bisphosphonates—may aggravate preexisting reflux disease and consequently potentiate cough. A good clinical investigation is necessary to differentiate drug-induced chronic cough from asthma. Determining and stopping the causative drug in etiology will be beneficial in both diagnosis and treatment. Spirometry also helps in diagnostic differentiation.

18. Tuberculosis

Tuberculosis (TB) is an infectious disease caused by *Mycobacterium tuberculosis* and other members of the *Mycobacterium tuberculosis* complex (MTBC) [69]. The disease resulted in 1.3 million fatalities in 2022 [70], and it is estimated that more than 31 million TB-related deaths will occur in the coming years. The lungs are the most affected organs [71]. However, the disease can also affect other sites such as the pleura, lymph nodes, abdomen, genitourinary system, skin, joints, bones, and meninges. The symptoms of pulmonary tuberculosis (PTB) are diverse and include, but are not limited to, persistent cough, hemoptysis, fatigue, weight loss, night sweats, and fever. It is important to note that these symptoms may be mild or even absent in the early stages of the disease. TB is a contagious disease. The primary method of transmission is through cough-generated aerosols. The progression of the disease from the point of transmission is influenced by a variety of factors, including environmental conditions, the viability of the microbial organism, and the immune response of the host. Sputum smear microscopy, radiological imaging, microbiological culture production, and molecular diagnostic methods can be used for disease diagnosis. Tuberculin skin tests and interferon gamma release tests are used for infection diagnosis [72].

TB treatment is carried out according to the drug resistance pattern observed in sputum culture results and national guidelines. Treatment is long-term and requires compliance and observation. Although TB shows respiratory symptoms, it can be easily distinguished from asthma both because the symptoms include a more productive cough and systemic findings (such as fever and fatigue) and because it is recognized radiographically. Although it may resemble asthma with mild respiratory symptoms in the early TB period, having a history of contact with the patient will be quite helpful in the distinction. Asthma and TB are completely different entities in terms of diagnosis and treatment approaches.

19. Conclusions

The clinical presentations of airway and parenchymal lung diseases may bear a resemblance to those of asthma, thereby resulting in diagnostic challenges. A comprehensive evaluation—including a detailed medical history, thorough physical examination, and appropriate laboratory and radiological investigations—is essential for accurate differentiation. Establishing a precise differential diagnosis is critical, as it directly influences therapeutic decision-making and prognostic outcomes for both asthma and the alternative conditions under consideration.

Acknowledgements

No funding information.

Conflict of interest

The authors declare no conflict of interest.

Author details

Guzin Ozden[1*] and Leyla Cevirme[2]

1 University of Health Sciences Adana City Training and Research Hospital, Adana, Turkey

2 Adana City Training and Research Hospital, Adana, Turkey

*Address all correspondence to: drkocamazguzin@hotmail.com

References

[1] Donaldson AM. Upper airway cough syndrome. Otolaryngologic Clinics of North America. 2023;**56**(1):147-155

[2] Morice AH et al. ERS guidelines on the diagnosis and treatment of chronic cough in adults and children. The European Respiratory Journal. 2 Jan 2020;**55**(1):1901136. DOI: 10.1183/13993003.01136-2019. Erratum in: European Respiratory Journal. 2020 Nov 19;56(5):1951136. DOI: 10.1183/13993003.51136-2019

[3] Rouadi PW et al. WAO—ARIA consensus on chronic cough: Executive summary. World Allergy Organization Journal. 2025;**18**(3):101034

[4] Global Initative For Asthma. Global Strategy for Asthma Management and Prevention. 2024. Available from: www.ginasthma.org

[5] Boyd M et al. Tracheobronchial foreign body aspiration in adults. Southern Medical Journal. 2009;**102**(2):171-174

[6] Yilmaz A et al. Occult bronchial foreign body aspiration in adults: Analysis of four cases. Respirology. 2004;**9**(4):561-563

[7] Bozkurt B et al. Universal definition and classification of heart failure: A report of the Heart Failure Society of America, Heart Failure Association of the European Society of Cardiology, Japanese Heart Failure Society and Writing Committee of the Universal Definition of Heart Failure: Endorsed by the Canadian Heart Failure Society, Heart Failure Association of India, Cardiac Society of Australia and New Zealand, and Chinese Heart Failure Association. European Journal of Heart Failure. 2021;**23**(3):352-380

[8] Halvorsen T et al. Inducible laryngeal obstruction: An official joint European Respiratory Society and European Laryngological Society statement. The European Respiratory Journal. 9 Sep 2017;**50**(3):1602221. DOI: 10.1183/13993003.02221-2016

[9] Leong P et al. Diagnosis of vocal cord dysfunction/inducible laryngeal obstruction: An International Delphi Consensus Study. The Journal of Allergy and Clinical Immunology. 2023;**152**(4):899-906

[10] Christensen PM et al. ERS/ELS/ACCP 2013 international consensus conference nomenclature on inducible laryngeal obstructions. European Respiratory Review. 2015;**24**(137):445-450

[11] Kanjanawasee D et al. Chronic cough management: Practical guidelines and PICO-based evidence for screening and investigation. Asian Pacific Journal of Allergy and Immunology. 2024;**42**(4):305-317

[12] Pfortmueller CA et al. Primary hyperventilation in the emergency department: A first overview. PLoS ONE. 2015;**10**(6):e0129562

[13] Hunt JF et al. Endogenous airway acidification. Implications for asthma pathophysiology. American Journal of Respiratory and Critical Care Medicine. 2000;**161**(3 Pt 1):694-699

[14] Eapen AA et al. Gastroesophageal reflux disease, laryngopharyngeal reflux, and vocal cord dysfunction/inducible laryngeal obstruction-overlapping conditions that affect asthma. The Journal of Allergy and Clinical Immunology. 2024;**154**(6):1369-1377

[15] White J, Dubey S. Eosinophilic granulomatosis with polyangiitis: A review. Autoimmunity Reviews. 2023;**22**(1):103219

[16] Masi AT et al. The American College of Rheumatology 1990 criteria for the classification of Churg-Strauss syndrome (allergic granulomatosis and angiitis). Arthritis and Rheumatism. 1990;**33**(8):1094-1100

[17] Moiseev S et al. International consensus on ANCA testing in eosinophilic granulomatosis with polyangiitis. American Journal of Respiratory and Critical Care Medicine. 25 Jun 2020. DOI: 10.1164/rccm.202005-1628SO. Epub ahead of print

[18] Matucci A et al. EGPA phenotyping: Not only ANCA, but also eosinophils. Biomedicine. 3 Mar 2023;**11**(3):776. DOI: 10.3390/biomedicines11030776

[19] Stanojevic S et al. ERS/ATS technical standard on interpretive strategies for routine lung function tests. The European Respiratory Journal. 13 Jul 2022;**60**(1):2101499. DOI: 10.1183/13993003.01499-2021

[20] Evans NJ et al. The incidence, duration, risk factors, and age-based variation of missed opportunities to diagnose pertussis: A population-based cohort study. Infection Control and Hospital Epidemiology. 2023;**44**(10):1629-1636

[21] Couzigou C, Flahault A. Is pertussis being considered as a cause of persistent cough among adults? European Journal of Epidemiology. 2003;**18**(10):1013-1015

[22] Centers for Disease Control and Prevention. Pertussis (Whooping Cough). Surveillance & Reporting. Available from: https://www.cdc.gov/pertussis/php/surveillance/?CDC_AAref_Val=https://www.cdc.gov/pertussis/surv-reporting.html [Accessed: July 13, 2024]

[23] Aliberti S et al. Criteria and definitions for the radiological and clinical diagnosis of bronchiectasis in adults for use in clinical trials: International consensus recommendations. The Lancet Respiratory Medicine. 2022;**10**(3):298-306

[24] Chalmers JD et al. Bronchiectasis. Nature Reviews Disease Primers. 2018;**4**(1):45

[25] Quint JK et al. Changes in the incidence, prevalence and mortality of bronchiectasis in the UK from 2004 to 2013: A population-based cohort study. The European Respiratory Journal. 2016;**47**(1):186-193

[26] Keir HR, Chalmers JD. Pathophysiology of bronchiectasis. Seminars in Respiratory and Critical Care Medicine. 2021;**42**(4):499-512

[27] Carpagnano GE et al. Severe uncontrolled asthma with bronchiectasis: A pilot study of an emerging phenotype that responds to mepolizumab. Journal of Asthma and Allergy. 2019;**12**:83-90

[28] Coman I et al. Bronchiectasis in severe asthma: Clinical features and outcomes. Annals of Allergy, Asthma & Immunology. 2018;**120**(4):409-413

[29] Polverino E et al. The overlap between bronchiectasis and chronic airway diseases: State of the art and future directions. The European Respiratory Journal. 15 Sep 2018;**52**(3):1800328. DOI: 10.1183/13993003.00328-2018

[30] Shoemark A et al. Characterization of eosinophilic bronchiectasis: A

European Multicohort Study. American Journal of Respiratory and Critical Care Medicine. 2022;**205**(8):894-902

[31] Oriano M et al. T2-high endotype and response to biological treatments in patients with bronchiectasis. Biomedicine. 2 Jul 2021;**9**(7):772. DOI: 10.3390/biomedicines9070772

[32] Mac Aogain M et al. Distinct "immunoallertypes" of disease and high frequencies of sensitization in non-cystic fibrosis bronchiectasis. American Journal of Respiratory and Critical Care Medicine. 2019;**199**(7):842-853

[33] Radovanovic D et al. A comprehensive approach to lung function in bronchiectasis. Respiratory Medicine. 2018;**145**:120-129

[34] Celli B et al. Definition and nomenclature of chronic obstructive pulmonary disease: Time for its revision. American Journal of Respiratory and Critical Care Medicine. 2022;**206**(11):1317-1325

[35] Sin DD et al. Air pollution and COPD: GOLD 2023 committee report. European Respiratory Journal. 11 May 2023;**61**(5):2202469. DOI: 10.1183/13993003.02469-2022

[36] Yang IA, Jenkins CR, Salvi SS. Chronic obstructive pulmonary disease in never-smokers: Risk factors, pathogenesis, and implications for prevention and treatment. The Lancet Respiratory Medicine. 2022;**10**(5):497-511

[37] Agusti A et al. Pathogenesis of chronic obstructive pulmonary disease: Understanding the contributions of gene-environment interactions across the lifespan. The Lancet Respiratory Medicine. 2022;**10**(5):512-524

[38] Venkatesan P. GOLD COPD report: 2025 update. The Lancet Respiratory Medicine. 2025;**13**(1):e7-e8

[39] Cosio BG et al. Defining the asthma-COPD overlap syndrome in a COPD cohort. Chest. 2016;**149**(1):45-52

[40] Barnes PJ. Asthma-COPD coexistence. The Journal of Allergy and Clinical Immunology. 2024;**154**(2):275-277

[41] Thomson NC. The role of smoking in asthma and chronic obstructive pulmonary disease overlap. Immunology and Allergy Clinics of North America. 2022;**42**(3):615-630

[42] Polverino F, Sin DD. Type 2 airway inflammation in COPD. The European Respiratory Journal. 28 May 2024;**63**(5):2400150. DOI: 10.1183/13993003.00150-2024

[43] Westafer LM, Long B, Gottlieb M. Managing pulmonary embolism. Annals of Emergency Medicine. 2023;**82**(3):394-402

[44] Konstantinides SV et al. ESC guidelines for the diagnosis and management of acute pulmonary embolism developed in collaboration with the European Respiratory Society (ERS): The task force for the diagnosis and management of acute pulmonary embolism of the European Society of Cardiology (ESC). The European Respiratory Journal. 9 Oct 2019;**54**(3):1901647. DOI: 10.1183/13993003.01647-2019

[45] Antoine MH, Mlika M. Interstitial lung disease 2023 Jul 31. In: StatPearls [Internet]. Treasure Island (FL): StatPearls Publishing; Jan 2025

[46] King TE Jr. Approach to the adult with interstitial lung disease: Clinical

evaluation. In: Flaherty KR, editor. Up to Date. Wolters Kluwer; 2024

[47] Martinez FJ, Flaherty K. Pulmonary function testing in idiopathic interstitial pneumonias. Proceedings of the American Thoracic Society. 2006;**3**(4):315-321

[48] Raghu G et al. Idiopathic pulmonary fibrosis (an update) and progressive pulmonary fibrosis in adults: An official ATS/ERS/JRS/ALAT clinical practice guideline. American Journal of Respiratory and Critical Care Medicine. 2022;**205**(9):e18-e47

[49] Sunman B et al. Current approach in the diagnosis and management of allergic bronchopulmonary Aspergillosis in children with cystic fibrosis. Frontiers in Pediatrics. 2020;**8**:582964

[50] Carter C et al. Real-world effectiveness of biologic therapy in allergic bronchopulmonary aspergillosis. The Journal of Allergy and Clinical Immunology. In Practice. May 2025;**13**(5):1094-1102.e1. DOI: 10.1016/j.jaip.2025.03.006. Epub 2025 Mar 13

[51] Praveen Akuthota PFW, Kauffman CA, Barnes PJ, Muller NL, editors. Clinical manifestations and diagnosis of allergic bronchopulmonary aspergillosis. In: Up to Date. Wolters Kluwer; 2024

[52] Maturu VN, Agarwal R. Prevalence of Aspergillus sensitization and allergic bronchopulmonary aspergillosis in cystic fibrosis: Systematic review and meta-analysis. Clinical and Experimental Allergy. 2015;**45**(12):1765-1778

[53] Agarwal R et al. Allergic bronchopulmonary aspergillosis: Review of literature and proposal of new diagnostic and classification criteria. Clinical and Experimental Allergy. 2013;**43**(8):850-873

[54] Agarwal R et al. Revised ISHAM-ABPA working group clinical practice guidelines for diagnosing, classifying and treating allergic bronchopulmonary aspergillosis/mycoses. The European Respiratory Journal. 4 Apr 2024;**63**(4):2400061. DOI: 10.1183/13993003.00061-2024

[55] Agarwal R et al. Long-term follow-up of allergic bronchopulmonary aspergillosis treated with glucocorticoids: A study of 182 subjects. Mycoses. 2023;**66**(11):953-959

[56] Agarwal R et al. Allergic bronchopulmonary aspergillosis. Clinics in Chest Medicine. 2022;**43**(1):99-125

[57] Muthu V et al. Allergic bronchopulmonary aspergillosis (ABPA) sans asthma: A distinct subset of ABPA with a lesser risk of exacerbation. Medical Mycology. 2020;**58**(2):260-263

[58] Eaton T et al. Allergic bronchopulmonary aspergillosis in the asthma clinic. A prospective evaluation of CT in the diagnostic algorithm. Chest. 2000;**118**(1):66-72

[59] Guo J, Garratt A, Hill A. Worldwide rates of diagnosis and effective treatment for cystic fibrosis. Journal of Cystic Fibrosis. 2022;**21**(3):456-462

[60] Burgel PR et al. The changing epidemiology of cystic fibrosis: The implications for adult care. Chest. 2023;**163**(1):89-99

[61] Cystic Fibrosis Foundation. 2023. Available from: https://www.cff.org/

[62] Marson FAL, Bertuzzo CS, Ribeiro JD. Classification of CFTR

mutation classes. The Lancet Respiratory Medicine. 2016;**4**(8):e37-e38

[63] Stewart C, Pepper MS. Cystic fibrosis on the African continent. Genetics in Medicine. 2016;**18**(7):653-662

[64] Yu E, Sankari A, Sharma S. Cystic fibrosis. In: StatPearls. Treasure Island (FL): StatPearls Publishing; Jan 2025

[65] Gilljam M et al. Clinical manifestations of cystic fibrosis among patients with diagnosis in adulthood. Chest. 2004;**126**(4):1215-1224

[66] Irwin RS et al. Classification of cough as a symptom in adults and management algorithms: CHEST guideline and expert panel report. Chest. 2018;**153**(1):196-209

[67] Tseng DS et al. Angiotensin-converting enzyme-related cough among Chinese-Americans. The American Journal of Medicine. 2010;**123**(2):183.e11-183.e15

[68] Ghouse J et al. Polygenic risk score for ACE-inhibitor-associated cough based on the discovery of new genetic loci. European Heart Journal. 2022;**43**(45):4707-4718

[69] Gagneux S. Ecology and evolution of *Mycobacterium tuberculosis*. Nature Reviews. Microbiology. 2018;**16**(4):202-213

[70] World Health Organization. Global Tuberculosis Report 2023. WHO; 2024. Available from: https://www.who.int/teams/global-programme-on-tuberculosis-and-lung-health/tb-reports/global-tuberculosis-report-2023

[71] Silva S et al. Economic impact of tuberculosis mortality in 120 countries and the cost of not achieving the sustainable development goals tuberculosis targets: A full-income analysis. The Lancet Global Health. 2021;**9**(10):e1372-e1379

[72] Bartolomeu-Goncalves G et al. Tuberculosis diagnosis: Current, ongoing, and future approaches. Diseases. 3 Sep 2024;**12**(9):202. DOI: 10.3390/diseases12090202